W9-BON-214

Hope Springs from Mended Places

Books by Diane M. Komp, M.D.:

A Window to Heaven:
     When Children See Life in Death
A Child Shall Lead Them: Lessons in Hope
     from Children with Cancer
Hope Springs from Mended Places:
     Images of Grace in the Shadows of Life

Hope Springs from Mended Places

Images of Grace
in the Shadows of Life

Diane M. Komp, M.D.

ZondervanPublishingHouse
Grand Rapids, Michigan

HarperSanFrancisco
San Francisco, California

Divisions of HarperCollins*Publishers*

Requests for information should be addressed to:
Zondervan Publishing House
Grand Rapids, Michigan 49530

Library of Congress Cataloging-in-Publication Data

Komp, Diane M.
    Hope Springs from Mended Places / Diane M. Komp.
        p.   cm.
    ISBN 0-310-43220-0 (alk. paper)
    1. Mothers—Religious life. 2. Sick children—Religous life. 3. Tumors in children—
Religious aspects—Christianity. 4. Suffering—Religious aspects—Christianity. 5.
Motherhood—Religious aspects—Christianity. 6. Mother and child. 7. Consolation. 8.
Women in the Bible. 9. Komp, Diane Me.
    I. Title.
    BV4529.K66   1993
    248.8'431—dc20   93-23699
                                                                                CIP

The *New Revised Standard Version* of the Bible, © 1990, by the National Council of
Churches of Christ in the United States of America, served as the basic biblical transla-
tion throughout. Minor changes in biblical texts were made for easier reading.

Edited by Lyn Cryderman
Interior design by Bob Hudson
Cover design by Jerry Fahselft
Cover illustration by Jerry Fahselt

94 95 96 97 98 99/❖DH/10 9 8 7 6 5 4 3 2 1

In memory of
Anna Florence Komp
and Adele Railey

Contents

Author's Preface   9

1. Rebekah's Twins   15

2. Mary Meets Martha   39

3. Tamar's Touch   59

4. Hannah's Exultation   71

5. Elena's Prayer   83

6. Hagar's Flight   99

7. Rahab's Crimson Cord   111

Author's Preface

In *A Window to Heaven*[1] I wrote about the spiritual experiences of children who would die from cancer. I told how my own life was changed by their witness. *In A Child Shall Lead Them*[2] I shared what these same children taught me about life and hope. What the children shared influenced the subsequent course of my life and career.

My original vision for this new book was to shift my focus from the children to their parents. Although centering on mothers' experiences, I am writing for all who care about children and their families. The shift will go ever further. Although I draw on my experiences with sick children, I want to point you past the illness to the ordinary and not-so-ordinary aspects of family life.

I've written about mothers before in the child-centered narratives of parents recorded in *Window* and *Child*. But who were these mothers before their children became my patients? Their lives did not begin with their child's diagnosis. They were shaped by their personal relationships as daughter, sister, wife, and friend—not by the diseases that brought their children into my world. Do I really know these mothers? Science alone does not offer all the hope that families need to mend.

The stories have the same setting as *Window* and *Child*—my practice as a specialist for blood diseases and cancer in children—but I reached for a "shared experience" to parallel the lives of the families I know. It was only in the Bible that I could find a frame of reference that related the families of my patients to all families. Rebekah and Rahab, Hannah and Hagar, Mary and Martha, and other biblical women suggested which stories to share. These biblical women serve as "hostesses" for the mothers I know and, with two exceptions, lent their names to my characters and the stories.[3]

I invite you to keep an open mind as you read, since your opinion of and familiarity with the Bible may be as much a disadvantage to you as an insider's track. I ask you to suspend any biases about the Bible —positive or negative—that you bring with you to these seven stories. Let the images, ancient and modern, come out of the shadows into full view before you draw your conclusions. I had to do that myself.

Let the characters in the book speak for themselves. Let them disturb you, point to your own broken places if you want to learn of hope and grace. You may find that the story you like best is the most removed from your own situation. It is the story that troubles you the most that I ask you to consider most carefully. It speaks of someone else's wounds, not your own.

Some of the biblical models suggested a particular ethnic focus or social structure to frame the modern story. The choices I made are in no way intended to suggest racial or cultural stereotypes or even represent typical families of sick children. I let the biblical story define which families from my practice to write about.

In *A Window to Heaven* I referred to the children as "reliable witnesses" and noted the directness with which they shared their thoughts, visions, prayers, and dreams. We adults would like to be reliable as well but are often reluctant to reveal our own stories. We do not share the children's lack of regret. Thus, a word about story form is in order.

The characters in these stories are blended composites from the thousands of families I've met during a career that spans thirty years and three major medical institutions in the United States and visiting professorships at a variety of European medical centers. None of these stories is a "straight line" following one family's journey. Names, places, and details have been changed wherever necessary to maintain the strictest confidentiality. Imagined elements and historical events have been added to enhance readability.

Although the main characters in this book are women, it is not my intention that this book be read only by women. Motherhood is important to *all* of us. Within these pages you will read of gracious women whose lives blessed all they touched, but you will also encounter tragic heroines who cry out for grace-filled solutions to ageless problems. Some of us—men and women—would like to believe that these troubling experiences have nothing to do with our own lives. That, my friend, would be a graceless exit from the reality of our own and the biblical world. Most of these families are just like yours and mine: in need of grace for strength to be made perfect in weakness.

It is my hope that these stories will encourage you to be a bearer of grace to all families, sharing in their suffering. And what you hear from me through these several witnesses, entrust to faithful people who will be able to teach others as well.[4]

Diane M. Komp
New Haven, Connecticut

Notes

1. Grand Rapids: Zondervan, 1992
2. Grand Rapids: Zondervan, 1993
3. Moses' mother's name was changed from Jochebed to Elena to better suit the ethnic context and avoid confusion with Jonadab, an essential villain in another piece.
4. 2 Timothy 2:1–3, adapted

1

Rebekah's Twins

When her time to give birth was at hand, there were twins in her womb. The first came out red, his whole body like a hairy mantle; so they named him Esau. Afterward his brother came out, with his hand gripping Esau's heel.

Genesis 24, 25

*T*he welcoming ceremony was about to begin. It took Becky longer than other mothers to move from the waiting area to an examining room. First, she must traverse our clinic gauntlet as all eyes converged on the peas from her proud pod.

At the nursing station, a spray of white dots on a dark blue background wiggled onto the scales. "Are you really Ruth or are you Leah?" Nurse Peggy pleaded with the child, not knowing if she was weighing the correct twin. Behind Peggy, an inverse set of dots, blue on white, giggled. The nurse groped for her eyeglasses, ceremoniously untangling them from her necklace of keys and bandage scissors. Clearer eyesight did not resolve her predicament, for she could not tell the girls apart.

Only one of the twins was my patient, but Peggy decided to weigh them both. She relished handing me a riddle with the chart: *Navy dots on white: 35 pounds; white dots on navy: 45 pounds.* Their mother always knew who was who, but not many other mortals shared Becky's certainty. Peggy counted herself among the ranks of mere mortals. In most ways, Ruth and Leah were indistinguishable, from the teasing gray eyes to the missing front teeth. But there was a consequential disparity: Only Ruth had leukemia.

It was easier to tell the girls apart when Ruth was going through the intensive part of her chemotherapy. Leah was the one with curly blonde hair. Ruth was the one who said, "If you're nice, I'll let you stroke my silky bald head." But now her hair is fully regrown. Now you have to wait for the dreaded pulse of prednisone for the scales and Ruth's chipmunk cheeks to tip off the difference. Doctors and nurses from other specialty clinics paused in their own activities to join the parade, as if they would miss a mitzvah if they failed to greet Ruth and Leah. I smiled myself at the mystery—that outsiders yearn to linger and comment. Unmitigated strangers feel entitled—nay, obligated—to gape at Mother Nature's miracle mirror. I chided myself for joining in the voyeurism. *They are two individuals,* I told myself, *not two halves of one child.* Each needs to be respected for who she is. But I missed Leah if she did not come with her sister, for there seemed to be something lost.

Joey's mother was in the clinic that particular day. Her own child, immersed in a Nintendo game, ignored her. "Who's Ruth, and who's Leah?" she queried. The girls sighed, refusing to enlighten their inquisitor. As long as there will be twins, there will be inquisitors. It was anyone's guess that day which was Leah and which was Ruth. When I walked in the room, I shook my head incredulously at the vision of frilly white panties before me. Ruth had swooped down to recover a fallen toy from the floor, offering the entire staff a ruffled peep show, encouraging my thoughts to wander home.

ﻌ   ﻌ   ﻌ

A painting hangs over my fireplace at home. In a lovely garden scene, watercolors shimmer in the freshness of summer sunshine. Hollyhocks sway in a mild breeze as if they are there to set the rhythm for two figures we see at work. Only the blossoms behold the children's faces. The artist leaves us to surmise what the snapdragons surely know. Little girls about the age of Ruth and Leah stand with their backs toward us. Twin sisters, they are pinning laundry onto a backyard clothesline. We see only silky pale-blonde hair, starched candy-stripe dresses, and white multi-layered frills peeking out from beneath. In the painting, one child bends from the waist, picking dolls' clothes out of a basket.

For many years this picture was a source of family controversy. It still is. Since you cannot see the faces, even those who allege inerrant discernment cannot say for certain which twin it is. My sister and I each contend that it is the other whose ruffled derriere salutes the spectator.

The watercolor was based on one of many prize-winning photos that my father took of us in our childhood. A grandaunt in Chicago was the artist who transformed our urban driveway into a country garden with the aroma of roses and Rinso White.

The painting hung prominently in my parents' home when we were children. Today it hangs in mine. As a child, I hated for people to see it. There was the inevitable question that followed, asked only of The Twins. Which one of us was bent over? Guests in our home never seemed to ask our parents. The dreaded question was always directed to The Twins.

When we were growing up, my sister and I weren't just Di and Marge. To the rest of the world, we were the Komp twins. Or, more simply, just The Twins.

ꝫ⁊   ꝫ⁊   ꝫ⁊

Becky greeted the other mothers in the chemo room. Once, she—and these other women—had had an identity apart from their children. But that seemed a different lifetime, long since discarded. Mornings like these, she huddled with other waiting women and the occasional father who brought his child. When it was "just girls" in the room, intimacies were shared as if they had known each other for their entire lives.

Becky would have preferred to marry right after college, but her parents prevailed on her to wait and take her time. She taught social studies for a few years at a junior-high school in the Bronx until she met a fellow teacher named Manny. He shared her dreams for a large family. After their honeymoon, she composed an undated letter of resignation, ready to offer it to the principal when she became pregnant. Weekends, she and Manny drove north of the city in search of a house large enough for all of her dreams.

Many of her Hunter College chums talked of waiting till they were firmly established in their careers before they began their families. Not Becky. Like her Grandma Selma, Becky imagined presiding over a houseful of children. Each year her hopes for a family dwindled and her teaching contract was renewed. Eventually, she stopped going to her college reunions. Even her friends who planned to wait were now immersed in parenting. Becky was pained by the exclusivity of their baby talk. Everywhere, there seemed to be a reminder of what she did not have. Even away from home. On the beach where they vacationed, she always noted the babies. Her husband was at a loss how to relieve his wife of her emptiness.

Eventually, Becky quit the school in the Bronx, and they moved to a small house in Cos Cob. She was about to sign a teaching contract for a school in Connecticut when she became pregnant. No longer barren, Becky gladly retired from the work world. She reinvested in her original dreams and commingled her own identity with that of her impending issue. Rebekah was to be the mother of twins!

Near the end of her pregnancy, Becky could hardly move. At night she lay in bed like a massive lump as she and Manny watched the late-night belly-war. Her husband tenderly stroked the spot where the last blow seemed to surface. "Hey, you guys in there!" he would call into her inverted navel. "It's time to go to sleep. You can pick up the battle tomorrow." Becky wondered what they thought they were competing for.

Mother and father were both exhausted from the nightly baby fistfights. When the twins weren't punching each other out, they were tap dancing on Becky's bladder. She was secretly relieved when they were born ahead of their due date.

Leah came easily and was the first to be born. But Ruth was a breech baby, bum first. Out of it all were born their new, unique identities. "Baby Girl A" and "Baby Girl B" metamorphosized into The Twins. And Rebekah became known as The Mother of The Twins.

She savored her new role in life. Becky felt unique, respected, admired, novel, proud. Her tiny daughters stared across her body when they nursed, their infant eyes trying so hard to converge on that other self. But when they cried, Becky imagined that they picked up their argument where they had left off *in utero*. Is it possible that two babies can sound louder than one plus one?

Manny nicknamed his wife "The Great Equalizer," as she spent all her energy trying to make sure neither child had more than the other. For the first three years her happiness was interrupted only by childish squabbles. It seemed that the harder she struggled to keep them equal, the more the children struggled to pull apart. Then, one day, Leah hit Ruth, and a nosebleed began that would not stop.

That was how the leukemia started. Both girls were there when I came to the Emergency Room late that night. Ruth lay like a silent slab of stone on the hospital gurney. Leah was screeching and scratching at her mother's face. Becky went with me to the treatment room when I did the test that confirmed their pediatrician's suspicion and her own worst fear. Ruth was so weak that she did not even struggle.

Leah remained with Manny, howling the whole time. "I want my mommy," she cried and was clearly heard through the closed door. This brutalized Becky more than any pain that Ruth might receive at my hand. She felt torn in half. Over the weeks to come, I noticed something unusual in their relationship. I'd dealt with dozens of pairs of twins as patients, but this was the first time I ever felt a tension between the two. Some cling closer to their twin than they do to their parents, unable to tolerate the briefest separation. But Ruth and Leah wanted to separate from each other, each tugging Becky in her own direction. In turn, Becky tried to pull and push them back toward each other. Their mother invested much of her energy into this grand-scale balancing act.

Once leukemia came into their home, Becky interpreted a simple sibling row as a risk to Ruth's life. When the inevitable squabble erupted, Leah was always questioned and usually blamed. Ruth relished her position as victim, first in her mother's concerns. As time passed, Leah became more sullen.

Her favorite line was, "It's not fair!" Frequently, it wasn't. Most of the major brouhahas occurred in private. For the masses, The Mother held court and The Twins held their tongues. They knew their mother's expectations. Both children came for every clinic visit. I suspected that Leah prized the attention more than Ruth. She certainly had less to suffer for the encounter. Only once did we take blood from her. Usually, she was there to entertain and be entertained.

Ruth's health returned quickly, and her visits became reasonably routine. Her treatment plan was for three years of chemotherapy, daily pills, and less-frequent shots. We had every reason to expect that she would be one of the fortunate children with acute lymphoblastic leukemia to survive.

Becky never shared my optimism. From the very beginning, she wanted to plan for a relapse. It was in this context that we drew blood from Leah, confirming her eligibility as a bone-marrow donor. Becky congratulated Leah. If Ruth relapsed, she would save her sister's life.

 è&   è&   è&

From time to time, Becky and I sat down together for tea and twin-talk. "Are you and your sister close?" she asked. Her question caught me off-guard. Most twin-mothers simply ask me if we still look alike.

"No, not really," I had to admit. "Sometimes I think that we're closer now than when we were younger. Perhaps because we live at a distance, the miles give us more room to breathe."

These conversations tended to be brief, but Becky never let me drop the subject without asking about my mother, what it was like for her to be The Mother of The Twins. My mother was an only child who wanted more than anything else to have a large family. She had great difficulty conceiving, and then only once did she become pregnant. In a way, God answered her heart's desire with the twin pregnancy. She didn't want to mother an only child. "But what was it *really* like for her?" Becky pushed. "Did she ever tell you?" Becky was asking not the mother but the daughter. Can a child ever truly speak for the mother, cut the cord, step back, and take a clearer, cleaner look?

My mother (who died more than twenty years ago) loved to talk about being a mother. While growing up, I heard her recite the details of her pregnancy many times over. These were the stories that I remember, the apotheosis of her blossoming double burden. Many of her stories began, "When you and your sister . . ." My mother loved being The Mother of The Twins.

❧   ❧   ❧

At our hospital all our little patients have rituals. Ruth and Leah were no different. When I entered the examining room, I was supposed to guess if the correct twin was sitting on the table. I never erred. I said that it was my powers as a twin that guided me. It was actually a slightly coarser turn to Ruth's curls when they regrew after chemotherapy. It took a clinically practiced eye to mark the difference. None of the other doctors shared my discernment. The Twins believed in the secret power of another twin. Sometimes I played along, dutifully examining Leah. I frowned when I palpated her belly, *hummmmmmmmmmmed* for the longest time when I auscultated her chest. "Okay, Ruth," I said, "there's something else I need to check. I know you're in a hurry today, so I'm not going to send you back to the lab. Just let me draw your blood right here and now."

Leah shrieked, Ruth squealed, and Becky dutifully reported that I had the wrong twin. Simultaneously both girls said, "Or did you know all along?" I simply grinned my omniscient twin-grin.

The twins were settled in together in the chemo room on a lounge chair watching *The Littlest Mermaid* when I walked with Becky to our kitchenette.

"What was it like for you growing up?" she asked, looking into her teacup. Was she a psychotherapist or the mother of one of my patients? I grubbed through old memories, unearthed something of that which she sought. On the Christmas Eve that came to mind, snow was falling.

ॐ ॐ ॐ

We lived in an old brownstone in Brooklyn then, not far from where Becky herself grew up. Many of the rooms railroad-carred into each other by a door through to the next room. I can't remember which room our private elves operated from. Whichever, on Christmas Eve, that room was off-limits to The Twins.

On childhood's most wondrous night of the year, I snuggled in bed listening for Christmas noises. I could hear Mom and Grandma chatting softly, accompanied by the whirring obbligato of an ancient Singer sewing machine. Their muffled voices moved in chanting waves over the surge and ebb of the next seam.

They would stay up all night, I imagined, sewing for us. Christmas morning, the world's best-dressed twin dolls sat under the tree, waiting for adoption. Our beaming elves stood by, waiting to see our faces when we saw the dresses they had made for us as well. After breakfast, they signaled Dad to put down the Brooklyn Eagle and get his camera gear. Mom and her mom were most content when they were working together. Grandma was an eighteen-year-old war widow when her only child was born. It was as if they had grown up together, two sisters. My grandmother had lived with us for as long as I could remember.

"Mom and Grandma were closer than Marge and I ever were," I told Becky. "I think closer than we will ever be." My grandmother outlived breast cancer, even metastases. Saddest for her, she even outlived her daughter. That was never her intention. I never heard her grieve. I simply felt her pain. Two years after my mother's death, I saw her smile return briefly when she held my sister's firstborn baby in her arms. A few days later, she didn't wake up.

ॐ   ॐ   ॐ

Becky dug some more, calling me abruptly back to the present. "Do you remember what your mother said when you and your sister fought?"

It isn't words that I remember. It was a profound sadness that Becky had dredged up. Mom didn't get angry very often. When we fought, I remember my mother's looking as if she had been mortally wounded.

ॐ   ॐ   ॐ

When Ruth and Leah started school, I was firm with Becky. Ruth was doing well, and her visits were fairly routine, but both children missed a day of school when the child with leukemia needed to be seen.

Becky and I skirmished over this school issue. There was a big chicken-pox epidemic one year, and she wanted to keep both girls out of school the entire year. I declined to sign a document for home schooling for the healthy child. I recommended that Leah be sent to school even if she got ahead of Ruth in her studies.

Unfortunately for her, it was Leah who developed chicken pox first. She was persona non grata in Cos Cob that week. Becky sent her into exile with Manny at an aunt's house on Long Island so that she would not further expose Ruth. Their mother acidly pointed out that Leah had been exposed on the school bus on one of the days she went to school and Ruth went alone to the clinic.

It was actually better for Ruth that we knew in advance exactly when she had been exposed. If both children had been exposed on the school bus without our knowledge, it could have been a lot worse. We were able to give Ruth a special gamma globulin in time. This medical clarification did not win points with Becky. There are times when logic goes unappreciated.

Poor Leah had a high fever and full-blown case, but Becky only visited her by phone. She was afraid that she would bring the virus home on her hands even if she wore surgical gloves when she touched her daughter. At home, she examined Ruth daily, looking for evidence of the scourge she feared. Three weeks after Leah, Ruth broke out with a grand total of two pocks. The gamma globulin had prevented a serious case. The rest was neutralized by an antiviral medicine. Ruth never even itched, but Leah returned from exile scabbed, scarred, and surly.

❧   ❧   ❧

There were little warning signals about Leah's wretchedness. The Twins were squabbling over the same toy one day when I walked into the examining room.

"I hate you!" Leah spat at her sister. "I wish you were dead."

I proposed a sibling support group for Leah, but Becky overruled my suggestion. She wanted a group where both children could be together. I wondered whether Leah would feel free in such a setting, or if the two would simply perform as The Twins. No matter how much my sister and I battled in private, we pulled together when we felt threatened. It was the two of us against the world. In public, we were always The Twins.

Ruth remained in remission, and her visits became less frequent. Then, unexpectedly, five years after she was first diagnosed, she relapsed. We set the plans in motion for a bone-marrow transplantation. Leah, her twin, was a perfect match.

The donation itself is done under general anesthesia because of the pain and length of the procedure. Although parents must give the legal consent, a child who is old enough to understand what it all means is invited to give her own assent. Thus, the team talked to Leah about what lay ahead.

None of us was prepared for what followed. Leah was terrified that she would go to sleep and not wake up. It didn't matter to her that that had never happened to any donor we knew. Social workers and child psychiatrists, determined to be her friends and advocates, all talked to Leah, but she remained firm and fearful.

It did not help in the least that I had shepherded countless families through difficult choices over the years. As many families of twins as I had dealt with, this was a novel dilemma. Becky was beside herself with anger. She could not bear to be in Leah's presence.

"She's a child," she thundered. "She doesn't know what she wants or doesn't want. Her sister could die while she enjoys a temper tantrum. We're their parents. Why can't we make that decision alone?"

I tried in vain to explain how important Leah's feelings were in all of this. Leah remained firm in her refusal. I imagined what it would have meant if it were my sister who might die. Sometimes we made casual jokes like, *I'll lend you a kidney if you lend me your bone marrow.* But that was the jesting of adult twins. I tried to remember what it might have been like when we were eight years old ourselves. I cannot believe that one of us would have refused.

❧   ❧   ❧

Once my sister nearly died. In our senior year in college, an inexperienced driver panicked in the fog. He let go of the steering wheel to shield his own face and hit a carful of student teachers head-on. My sister was one of them, riding in the suicide seat that day. She went through the windshield.

It was a Thanksgiving weekend when I caught a ride to far-off Indiana. We had agreed on separate colleges, almost a thousand miles apart. I remember seeing her bandaged face and newly rewired jaw. I can visualize the hospital chapel where I wept and prayed (I've never told her that). If worse had come to worst, I would never have refused to save her life. I may not have found the words, but I surely would have found the deed.

୬ଈ   ୬ଈ   ୬ଈ

Sibling rivalry, parental favoritism—these are common parts of family life but not ordinarily matters of life and death. Usually, the matter of bone-marrow donation is a voluntary act of a consenting adult, but this case involved two minor children. No matter what drama ruled their private lives, the medical staff had to ensure that both children's needs and rights were protected.

I tried talking to Leah without pressuring her, twin to twin. Her resentment was deep-seated. Leah was certain that Becky would sacrifice her for Ruth. Ever since her sister became ill, the child was aware of her mother's expectations. She recited them like a venomous litany. Leah believed that her mother loved her sister more. Leah interpreted Becky's efforts to restore parity as gross inequity.

My heart went out to the child we could not seem to help. The first steps toward the transplant needed to be set in motion long before we knew if it would ever actually happen. Unknown to Becky, this time of preparation turned into years in which Leah felt robbed of her birthright.

But as things turned out, Leah experienced all the pressure of deciding without ever having to donate. Ruth wasn't responding to chemotherapy and remained in the hospital, suffering one grim infection after another. Leukemic cells continued to grow through the most effective chemotherapy we knew. She wasn't going to survive long enough to receive anyone's marrow.

We reached the point where the institution of hospice home care would have been an appropriate choice. This was a bitter burden for Becky. She counted on the transplant and refused to consider withdrawing intensive chemotherapy. I lamented for the child who was confined to a hospital bed rather than liberated for her final days at home. I asked Becky if Leah wanted to come to visit her sister. I hadn't seen her in more than a week. Their mother's eyes filled with tears.

"It's not fair," she mourned. "All I ever wanted to be was the mother of twins. If Ruth dies ..." She folded into my arms as we both struggled for words.

"You will always be The Mother of the Twins," I told her. "If they had both survived, someday they would have moved out of your home. Whether it be to college, or to live with husbands, the day would have come when all you would have at home is your memories. Even if the time you've had was shorter than you had expected, no one can take that away from you."

Becky moved to the windowsill, looking out as she spoke. "I know this sounds silly," she continued, "but I won't be special anymore. As the mother of twins I felt unique." She turned back toward me, gasping, "Save my daughter!" Her gasp dissolved into a sob.

"I wish to God I could save her, Becky." *How many times have I said those words?* "But whether Ruth lives or dies, you are unique. Each of us is. Even Ruth and even Leah. It's a paradox."

"Is that what this twin business is?" she asked. "A paradox?"

Yes, perhaps, I thought. *Paradox is the only word that seems to make sense.*

ﻌ ﻌ ﻌ

On Friday evening, Ruth lay dying. "The time has come to ask her what will make her happiest," I told Becky. The child asked to see her sister, and Manny brought her there.

The children didn't speak to each other. Leah simply crawled into the bed with Ruth, each folded toward the other. It was as if they had womb-work left to do. I never heard them speak a word.

Manny and Becky stood there on that Shabbat evening, blessing Ruth and Leah. *May God bless you and protect you. May God look your way and be gracious to you. May God favor you and bring you peace.* Manny held his wife as the twins held each other, until Ruth died. Then Becky climbed into the bed and held both her daughters, one cradled in each arm. And their father embraced them all.

It was two years later that I heard a timid tap on my office door and turned to find Leah. Our sibling support group was meeting that afternoon. She had asked Becky if she could come.

"What a wonderful surprise!" I said, opening the door wide. Becky signaled that she was going to call on our social worker while her daughter visited with me. Leah sat down in a chair, pulled it close to mine.

She looked around my office—a child-friendly place. I'm very proud of the love-gifts that fill my work space. There are children's paintings on every wall, each with a wonderful story. It was something on my desk that caught her attention, caused her to stand, reach, bring it closer. It was a silver-framed photo of two young boys. "Are they your sons or your sister's?" she asked. Most people would have assumed that the boys were mine.

"That's Mitch and Scotty. They're my sister's boys."

She looked around my desk for another picture and did not find what she sought. "Is your sister still alive?" she asked, a ten-year-old child who took nothing for granted! I reassured her that Marge was alive and well.

"Do you and your sister still look like twins?" she wondered, relaxing back into the chair, still examining the photo of my nephews.

"No, not really," I admitted. "I guess we could if we didn't fool around with our hair color and our weight didn't go up and down at different times. But we have a lot of the same mannerisms. Mitch and Scotty notice that.

"When they were younger," I remembered, "the boys used to shake their heads and say, 'It's not just that you look like Mommy!'" Leah giggled, realizing that the twin business can go on for a lifetime. And beyond.

"Are you and your sister close?" She was Becky's daughter!

"I don't think you could really say that, Leah. It wasn't always fun for us to be twins. In fact, there were times when it was downright hard." She nodded wisely. She seemed so young to be struggling with thoughts that were only feelings for me at her age. She picked up another picture off my desk. "Is that your mother?" She had located the other Mother of The Twins. "Did she make you dress alike?" she asked. You'd better believe it!

My sister and I finally rebelled in high school, one leaving the house earlier in the morning so that Mom wouldn't see that we weren't dressed alike. Strange— now we buy each other identical dresses. "It was hard for me to be a twin," Leah said. "Now it's even harder not to be. But I think it's harder for Mommy than for me." The child rose from her chair, walked to the window. "Sometimes I wonder whether Mommy can love just me," she said sadly.

"I'm sure she can, Leah," I offered. "But for your mom, being The Mother of The Twins was what made her feel special. In a way, you and your mom face the same struggle. When you're a twin, you're unique because there aren't many other twins around." I was thinking out loud again. "But then you're not unique, because there's another one just like you. And your mom has the same struggle."

I didn't know if the child would understand me, but I needed to work it out for myself. She turned from the window and laced her arms around my neck from behind. I was grateful for the small, warm hands, the soft reminder that I was not alone.

"It's sad," I told her, "but nobody much treats moms as special." It was not just Becky's face that filled a mother-sized space in my heart but the portrait of every woman who has come back to this office after a child's death, drawn back to a place where she was treated with respect, blessed for simply being who she was. A mother. *Honor thy mother that thy days may be long in the land.* Perhaps, if we truly honored mothers, blessed them, the Beckys of this world would not feel that something more than their child had died.

I rose from my chair and took the child in my arms, winding down my monologue on twinnery. Leah was no longer the three-year-old I first met. Nor the eight-year-old I knew when her sister died. She was almost a young woman. Someday she, too, may be a mother. I hope so.

"Leah, you are one of the most special women I've ever met in my entire life." I was telling the truth. "In some way, Ruth will always be part of you. It's almost as if I can hear her saying, *Blessings on you, my sister. I will always be with you, but I want you to be free to be you. Peace, my dear sister.*"

She lingered for a while in my arms. Then, she was ready to go. With a final glance at a painting on my office wall, she added, "The next time I come, I'll bring you one of my drawings." With that benediction, she withdrew from my office.

I walked to the office door and saw her farther on down the hall. She was standing arm in arm with Becky, talking to one of the nurses.

"Did I ever tell you how special my mom is?" the child asked the nurse, blessing her mother. "My mom is absolutely one of a kind."

Becky drew her daughter to her as they walked out together.

2

Mary Meets Martha

As they went on their way, Jesus came to a certain village, where a woman named Martha welcomed him into her home. She had a sister named Mary, who sat at the Lord's feet and listened to what he was saying.

Luke 10

I never worried about my clinic schedule's starting on time if Teddy Campbell's name was on the list. His mother always asked for the earliest possible appointment of the day. Long before the receptionist arrived, she and Teddy were there in the waiting area.

Martha wanted to be the first in line when the lab opened and the blood-drawing team looked for the first patient. Just fifteen minutes later, all the other patients would start drifting into the lab. It would be an hour before the full results for any of them would be known.

When I entered the examining room, Martha greeted me with Teddy's completed blood report. The day's results were already recorded in a notebook she had kept ever since Teddy's treatment began. With each new rotation of medical students, I must teach them how to interpret those numbers. Martha learned to make the calculations the day her son's treatment began. That's the way I like my days to begin.

At first, our techs refused to give reports to a parent for fear that we doctors would disapprove. But it wasn't worth the effort to argue with Martha week after week. For her peace of mind, she must have all the blood counts before she could leave for home. For her, there was worth in these values, consolation that could be quantified. And I had to admit that her exigency sped up my work day. When I couldn't find Teddy's medical chart, I would beg a peek at Martha's flow sheets.

When Mary Bonito finally gets to clinic with Sarah, the nurses are always glancing at the clock, sharing knowing looks. There is no way they can start up the baby's chemotherapy and still get to lunch themselves. Every week Mary asks for the latest possible appointment, but she never seems to make even that on time. A nurse comes to the doctor's conference room and begs me to talk to Mary again about punctuality.

Mary's stories don't vary much. She waited with her oldest son for the school bus, which, as usual, was late. Then, at the baby-sitter's house, there was a tearful farewell scene with her preschooler. Both boys have been afraid to leave Mary's side since Sarah was first admitted to the hospital. Mary wants them to know that she will always be there for them as well as their little sister.

The doctors for the next speciality clinic come drifting into the conference room, meaning to displace me as their own clinic is about to begin. "Why do your clinics always seem to run so late?" they grouch.

ॐ   ॐ   ॐ

Nine-year-old Teddy and nine-month-old Sarah have the same disease. They came to us on the very same day, both suffering from a highly lethal form of neuroblastoma. Even their chemotherapy was the same. But their mothers were as different as midnight and daybreak.

Martha keeps in regular touch with parents at three other major treatment centers, comparing notes on treatment protocols. She shares with them what she learns from Teddy's doctors about the newest research. She asks other mothers about doses of the drugs their children receive so that she can enter it into her records.

The only mothers that Mary seeks out are those in the chemo room and the parents' support group. The medical details hold no import for her. Mostly, she concerns herself with how the other moms are doing, whether their children are happy.

Sarah and Teddy became ill at the same time and came to the same hospital. There the similarity seems to end, because Mary and Martha are as different as a fast and a feast.

When Teddy was born, Martha and Roger were ready. The young couple waited until they were financially secure before they started their family. They owned their first home, fully furnished. Everything—even Teddy—had been planned.

Roger liked his life in order, and Martha provided that order single-handedly. The other men in the office joked that their wives were more familiar with Montel Williams than Mr. Clean. Roger's buddies grumbled about the wages paid the latest maid. Martha's husband would never have to pay for a housekeeper. There was no one here on earth who could meet his wife's expectations. He had married a Lysol Lil who hoovered the floors twice a day. Nothing in their home was out of place.

The birth of their second child three years after Teddy brought a brief moment of disorder into the otherwise perfectly run household. Martha recovered quickly, brought all again into order. There was further slight discord when her sister came to help with Teddy, while Martha cared for the new baby.

The visit was shorter than originally scheduled. Martha's sister, Janet, liked to sit down after dinner. She would relax rather than immediately jump up to do the dishes. But Martha liked to load the dishwasher even before dessert was served. Roger had no grievance with sploshing while he was eating. It was dinner music for an antiseptic household.

The sisters' concepts of housekeeping didn't mesh. Janet felt she was there to assist, not to be converted. She left after three days, but no one really missed her for Martha could manage by herself.

Mary and Pete didn't plan her pregnancies. Their children just happily happened. Sarah was their third in six years, the baby of the family and the only girl. By the time little Sarah arrived, cheery mayhem had ruled their home for so long that Pete could not remember the last time he had seen an uncluttered house.

When guests appeared at the door, major obstacles were removed from the living-room floor. Someone briefly checked under sofa pillows to ensure that the dog hadn't buried any of his biscuits there. Humphrey waxed indignant if a visitor sat too close to his treasure trove. Naïve guests sometimes found themselves jowl-to-jowl with a pouting basset hound.

Pete and the animal came to the marriage together, two happy ex-bachelors. With two little ones in Pampers, Humphrey had his employments. Nose a-twitch, he prowled after rug-rats, sniffing and snitching, fixing on terminal targets until change was transacted. Then Humphrey trailed all the way to the diaper pail (chained shut to keep him out).

With each successive pregnancy, Pete seemed to pick up momentum when other men might find the novelty was wearing off. By the time Mary gave birth to Sarah, he and the other ex-bachelor had taken over the household. Pete placed the dirty dishes in the refrigerator, reasoning that it would control microbial overgrowth until he was ready to wash them. A handheld Dust Buster sufficed to suck the crumbs off the kitchen floor. Humphrey's tongue followed Pete's hand, slicking the linoleum to a high polish.

Mary's merry men curled up after supper to watch football on the tube. Humphrey's rump and Pete's lap pillowed the children's heads. By halftime, all four were snoring in concert. Mary's mother came a few days later, rescuing the family from the Pizza Taxi.

Pete never seemed to tire of the wonder of a newborn's entry into life. When the new mom came home from the hospital, he brought her breakfast in bed. He raced home from work in the middle of the day to watch his wife breast-feed his new daughter. He overstayed his lunch hour many a day, for Pete was a happy man.

かな かな かな

For Teddy, the illness began with an aching in his bones that kept him awake at night. Martha rocked him in her arms and sang to him. Nothing she could do seemed to help. The first pediatrician called it "growing pains." There was nothing to prescribe other than Tylenol. Martha had already tried that and begged for something stronger. The child was not a complainer. It was not like him to cry out in the night.

She changed doctors. The second pediatrician suggested arthritis as the diagnosis. Martha became frantic as her son became sicker and she received no answer that helped.

Teddy lost three pounds the last week before he came to us. The child was unable to eat by day. He cried in his sleep at night. Roger became irritable from the loss of sleep. He was easy to get along with when his life was in order, but he had low tolerance for disorder. Their entire married life, Martha had always been able to keep perfect order for them both. This was the first time that everything wasn't in her control.

Annabelle stopped by one day for coffee and found Martha hysterical in her own kitchen, repeating to herself, "Stay calm. Keep in control. Don't lose it." Her neighbor touched her hand, but Martha pulled away abruptly.

"No, I'm okay. I just didn't get very much sleep last night. Teddy seems so sick, and none of the doctors seems to know what's going on." It was then that Teddy cried out in such agony that Martha flew up the stairs, sobbing.

"I'm taking you to the Emergency Room, right now," Annabelle said and headed next door to get her car keys. It was there that Martha first heard the terrible word.

The pediatrician who examined Teddy took her to Radiology so that she could see the X-ray film for herself. On a back-lit view box, she saw white shadows on black. They meant nothing to her.

"Do you see, here and here?" he asked, pointing to what seemed like thigh bones. It was Teddy's legs they had photographed. "This should be all white, but the bones look moth-eaten, both legs."

He flipped a switch, lighting the next panel. More shadows, this time of the boy's body. "And here, on the belly films. This white area shouldn't be there. This is what's causing his pain. We think it's a tumor, a form of cancer."

Cancer! It was then that Martha knew that if Teddy would survive—if she would survive—she must get control of herself. Of all times in her life, this was the most important time that she be in control.

෨   ෨   ෨

She was bathing the baby one day when Mary noticed the little bump. It was a bluish mound under Sarah's skin, like a lump on a blueberry muffin. Then she noticed several other spots, all the same. They just weren't there a day before.

"Hon, would you come and look at this?" she called. Pete came into the baby's room and looked where Mary pointed. He didn't know what to think.

"Why don't you call Dr. Friedman? She'll know if it's anything important." So Mary called, and her pediatrician suggested an early appointment for the next morning. *Better to check it out,* the doctor said. *Hard to say over the phone.* But the baby was happy and fed well, so Mary was not particularly worried.

"Do you want me to take the day off and go with you?" Pete offered. She thought it sweet of him, but Mary declined. He had already missed so much work when the baby was born.

She went to the pediatrician's office by herself that day. As soon as Naomi Friedman saw the blue lumps under the skin, she frowned and started to probe around the rest of Sarah. She examined her for a long time, feeling deep in her abdomen.

"Mary, it's good that you noticed these so fast. That's always good. But that's not all that there is. There's a mass deep in her belly, near her kidney that I can feel."

"Mass? Are you talking about cancer?"

"Possibly. First I want to do a few tests in our lab. But then I'll be sending you over to the university hospital. Would you like me to call Pete? Do you want him to be there when we talk?"

"Yes, thank you." She held Sarah and nursed her while waiting for Pete. The baby nipped at Mary's breast playfully, not seeming to know there was anything wrong as her mother began to pray.

When Pete arrived, they drove together to the hospital. It was in the elevator to the children's floor that Mary first met Martha. On the same day that Teddy started his treatment on the school-age ward, baby Sarah began the fight for her life.

સ⬥   સ⬥   સ⬥

The six months of treatment began. One of the nurses came into the conference room to talk to me. "You need to talk to Mary. All the other mothers have learned to do the catheter care, but she seems to be on another planet. I don't think she is ever going to get it."

We had progressed so much in the treatment of these children that we had passed on much of the daily care to the mothers. Most of them, like Martha, seemed to like the responsibility. I went (as ordered) but heard another voice inside the room. I waited in the hall.

"I don't know why they expect that every mother will be Dr. Mom overnight," Mary's voice could be heard through the open door. "I'm just plain mom and never pretended to be anything else." She was talking to Martha.

"Here, let me show you how I do it," Martha offered. She set up the dressing kit very professionally and then showed Mary her personal little tricks.

"Well, maybe I can." Mary was encouraged.

"You've got it! See, I told you that you could do it," Martha triumphed.

When I heard her voice in the room, I knew that I did not need talk to Mary. Martha was our parent pro. Mary would get it now. Twice Martha visited her at home, and they changed the dressing together. Martha seemed to be a natural when it came to working our things out.

爨   爨   爨

Six months later, Teddy and Sarah were in the chemo room at the same time. "I don't know what the holdup is," Martha worried to the nurse. "His counts were ready long ago. Why isn't the chemo here yet?"

"That's okay, Mom," interjected Teddy, mesmerized by a Ninja Turtle video he was watching. "I'm in no hurry."

"I wish you wouldn't watch that trash," Martha complained to her son. "I brought tapes for you to listen to on your Walkman. Try to visualize your white cells fighting your tumor. Think positive thoughts."

"Sometimes it's not very positive having cancer, Mom. In fact, it stinks!" He still looked like an ordinary little boy, but in six months, Teddy seemed to have aged sixty years.

"Now if you could just channel all that anger against your tumor, you just might beat it," Martha scolded him.

"The only channel I'm interested in today is the Disney Channel. Let's not get too serious about all this business, Mom. You're not the one getting the chemo. This chemo is the best that anyone has. If it doesn't work, it's nobody's fault. It's not your fault or mine."

That was the point at which I had walked into the room. It was Teddy's last few words that caught my attention. *Nobody's fault.* I was worried about Martha. She held herself responsible for the lives and living of all she loved.

If the tumor came back, would she see it as her fault for not having researched enough? Or Teddy's fault because he preferred Ninja dudes to guided imagery? Or my fault because everyone likes to blame doctors today? Most likely, she would blame herself.

The problem was that the tumor *was* back. The reason for the delay in his chemo was a call I placed to the clinic from the Radiology Department. I told the nurse to hold the drugs. Despite everything we had offered Teddy, despite everything Martha had done, the neuroblastoma was back.

ᏋᏛ   ᏋᏛ   ᏋᏛ

In bed that night, Pete sensed Mary's preoccupation. "Is something the matter, Hon? You seem to be in another world. Did something happen with Sarah today at the hospital?"

"It isn't Sarah. It's Teddy." She put down her prayer journal on the bedside table. For six months, every night, she had prayed over every family she met in our clinic. Each family had its own page. She was not the type to make a big issue of her beliefs publicly, but she was faithful in her private commitment to everyone she met.

"His tumor is back," Mary continued. "His mom took the news very hard. Teddy had to reassure Martha, promise her that he would fight it. I heard him talking to Dr. Komp afterward. He already knew before the X-ray was taken. All week he's been having pain in his arm. He knew what it meant, but he didn't say anything."

"There's nothing you can do for Martha," Pete interjected.

"She's talking about taking Teddy to another cancer center for an experimental treatment she heard about from another mother. She didn't even tell the doctors that. I heard her telling Teddy. The poor kid said, 'But Mom, I like it here. These people are my friends.' She blew up at him, 'This is your life we're talking about!' It wasn't a very pleasant scene.

"It's the strangest thing." Mary nestled to her husband, comforted by the familiar. "I had the feeling that she was angry with me, as if it were my fault. She asked me how Sarah is doing, and I was afraid to tell her that we had a good report.

"They started the same time, Sarah and Teddy. Martha had learned everything possible about neuroblastoma, followed his blood counts so carefully. And I never did any of that and Sarah is okay."

"Seems to me," said Pete, pulling her closer to him, "that there was a time that you accepted the responsibility for everything and everybody. When we first met, the entire Holocaust was your fault because your Uncle Hugo served in the *Luftwaffe*. Then it was the American Indians. They buried your heart at Wounded Knee."

Mary poked him in the ribs, "Come on! I don't even take the responsibility for your dirty socks anymore. I just leave them where you throw them until you trip over them or can't find any more to wear.

"But it's hard for someone like Martha," Mary continued. "She's always been so efficient and competent. Her house was always immaculate. Since Teddy's been sick, she realizes that she can't take care of the whole world alone, not even the people close to her."

"What's happening with her and Roger?" Pete asked. "I met him once at Candlelighters, and we just didn't connect. I was able to find something in common with all the other men, but Rog and I didn't seem to have mutual interests. He seemed to hide himself in his work when Teddy got sick. He just wanted to talk about insurance claims."

Pete's comment reminded Mary of a new concern. "Today when Dr. Komp told her the news, I asked Martha if she wanted to call Roger. I offered to stay with Teddy while she called. She just shook her head and got teary-eyed. She and Teddy looked at each other funny."

꒰ꕤ   ꒰ꕤ   ꒰ꕤ

The first week after his relapse, Teddy got by with simple Tylenol, but then the pain accelerated and he reached the point he was at when the tumor was first found. Martha heard him crying in the night, awakening from her sleep. She turned toward Roger, forgetting that he was gone. It had been two months since he lived at home with them.

What hurt most was learning that Roger was already involved with another woman before Teddy became sick. As long as he had his perfect home and orderly life, he could tolerate his marriage. But cancer had changed all that, and he did not like the change. He blamed it all on Martha. This other relationship was undemanding, far simpler.

Martha went to Teddy's room and measured out the morphine to give him. She rocked him as it started to work its effect. She fell asleep with her child in her arms.

There was a knock at the door, late that night. The dream was so real that Martha told herself in her dream that this was no dream. She got up—in her dream—and went down to answer the door. At her front door was a carpenter, dressed in bib overalls with tools hanging from his waist. He held a lantern that was so bright that he seemed surrounded by light. But the light did not blind Martha nor hurt her eyes.

The carpenter told Martha that her house needed fixing and that he had come to repair it. She needed not fear, for he would put her house in order. She should simply rest. In this dream that seemed no dream, Martha surrendered herself to the deep, peaceful gift of sleep. In the morning, she woke with Teddy in her arms.

The child whimpered slightly when she touched him. She reached for another dose of morphine as she kissed him on the forehead. "It's okay, Teddy," she murmured. "We're going to the hospital. Like you said, they're your friends there. They'll take care of the pain."

The next few days were crisis days for Teddy. Despite the morphine and chemotherapy, the tumor seemed to be progressing. He started bleeding from his stomach, and we couldn't seem to stop it. We transferred him to Intensive Care. The clinic nurses came to visit him there. He and Martha were among their favorites.

All the other mothers knew about Teddy. There is always a slight sense of guilt when your own child is doing well and another woman's son is dying, but everyone understood the common pain of belonging to the same family.

But there was another overwhelming pain that Martha must face in her unextended family. Teddy's hospitalization brought her and Roger back into daily contact. Because of the child that they both loved, they could not avoid facing each other across Teddy's bed. Together, they began to face that other pain.

❧　❧　❧

Mary was there with Sarah as well the day that Teddy went to the ICU. Sarah was to be admitted for her last course of chemotherapy. A "coming off" party had been planned for the final day, a rite of passage.

When Sarah was settled in, Mary went to the Hunan Wok and brought food back to the ICU. Mary and Martha sat there silently eating, not even tasting the spicy meat. It was Martha who broke the silence in an uneven staccato.

"Do you know how much I resented you all these months? I'm ashamed to admit it. I even thought I hated you."

"Hush," said Mary, taking Martha into her arms. "You didn't really mean it. I know that." The tears were overflowing, and Martha let them wash out her pain.

"The worst day of all was the day that Teddy relapsed. I hated you that you never seemed to work at being the mother of a child with cancer and yet Sarah was doing well. She was even going to finish up her chemotherapy. How I hated you!"

Mary held Martha in her arms and rocked with her. I found them there together an hour later. There was unity and symmetry all at once in the pose, for were they not each a part of the other, a member of every mother? And both a part of me.

৯৯   ৯৯   ৯৯

Late that night I returned to see a new patient in the Emergency Room. This child and her family were now settled in on the school-age floor. Tomorrow would be a big day for them and me. Before leaving for home, I stopped by to check on the rest of my brood.

Sarah slept quietly in her crib, Mary bedded down beside her. She was four days away from completing her treatment. Teddy also slept peacefully in the ICU, a grinning Garfield enfolded in his arms. In the side room where parents hold vigil, I found Martha and Roger, woven together, sleeping on a single cot.

I closed the door quietly to head home. Mary's daughter was on the homestretch. Martha's son was stable. And there were only a few hours left for me to sleep before the new day would begin.

3

Tamar's Touch

Tamar put ashes on her head, and tore the long robe that she was wearing; she put her hand on her head, and went away crying aloud as she went. Tamar remained, a desolate woman, in her brother Absalom's house.

2 Samuel 13

*T*oday some might call Carter Lowell a nerd. A longish mane spilled over his horn-rimmed glasses when he concentrated, forming a blond blind. Significant passages of his textbooks were punctuated by a sideways whiplash, a toss of head and neck to clear his vision. Book-bent was the common posture of this passionate scholar I knew years ago.

Although his school did not encourage accelerated progression, Carter had already skipped two grades by the time he reached the seventh. He was intrigued by the physical sciences. There was a lab in the corner of his bedroom filled with beakers and Bunsen burners, flasks and flames. He continued to experiment long past school hours. Excellent! That was one of Carter's favorite phrases.

The boy was not one of those family surprises, more brilliant than his forebears. Both his parents had earned advanced degrees from prestigious institutions. He was clearly their child.

Carter was conceived when his mother was in graduate school. The boy's father was a post doc who was one of her laboratory teaching assistants. Married to another woman, he returned to England with his wife when the boy was born.

ᘔ&ᘔ&ᘔ&

When the nurse first handed the newborn baby to her, Tamara was afraid to touch him for fear that he would break. He was so tiny! She was so inexperienced. Tamara dropped out of grad school to move back with her parents and care for the child. Carter never knew his father.

Eventually she went back to complete her degree, and by the time I met her, Tamara Lowell was a well-established research scientist. The boy grew up mostly in the care of his grandparents.

There was a spirit in the lad that seemed alien in that particular family. He often felt as if he was a disappointment to them, especially to his mother. He didn't know how to please her. There was a warmth in Carter that was missing in his mother, an anticipation that something exciting might happen when you meet ordinary people.

Carter Lowell followed a solitary path. He walked alone to school each day. He ate alone in the lunchroom; he joined the math team rather than take up a sport. He didn't have a girlfriend, nor had he ever attended a school dance. Carter excelled in academics but lived on the fringes of teenage society. Younger than his classmates by two years, he had no real chums at school. To them, Carter seemed somewhat pompous. The poor kid was simply so enthusiastic about learning that he had no discernment of when to remain silent in the presence of dolts. At sixteen, his passion was for Bach, not rock.

ॐ   ॐ   ॐ

It was a distracting pain in his shoulder that brought Carter to my office. The X-rays confirmed his family doctor's suspicion of a bone tumor. In all my years of practice, I've never had a conversation with a mother like that first session when I told Dr. Lowell that Carter had cancer.

With anger flashing in her eyes, Tamara raged, "We don't believe in God!" At that point in my life, neither did I, but there was such a hatred in her voice that I took sharp notice. I disbelieved quietly. There was a chilling intonation to Tamara's denunciation. This was her first thought when I told her that her son had cancer.

In those days, few teenagers with Ewing's sarcoma survived. Yet there were patients outliving our gloom-and-doom talk every day. I wanted to talk about treatment. Tamara wanted to talk about her son's death, there in that first meeting.

"How do patients with this tumor usually die?" she asked as her son listened, tears running down his face. I could not believe what I was hearing.

"It's possible that Carter may not die from this at all," I said. "We have treatment to offer. He may kick it rather than succumb to it."

"There won't be a service," his mother continued. "Not even an obituary in the papers. There is no life after death." It was at that point that I realized that I had never before met a parent of a child with cancer who actually claimed to be an atheist.

I asked about the boy's father, if he would be coming to see his son. The father, she said, was not a factor in his life and would hardly be a help in his death.

※ ※ ※

Months into his treatment, Carter's English teacher noticed a constant sadness and asked if he would like to talk to a counselor. In a brief conversation, the school psychologist learned enough to alarm him. He called Tamara to suggest formal therapy. The notion was hostilely rejected. The boy simply lacked discipline, she said. His grandfather would speak to him.

His grandfather did talk to him once, during early puberty when Carter began to masturbate compulsively. He threatened to cut off both the boy's hands if he ever did it again.

Eventually, Carter's sadness worked its way to the surface. He stole a car and crashed it into a telephone pole, nearly killing himself in the process. The juvenile court set psychotherapy as a condition for probation. Tamara had no other choice.

ɜ⚫ ɜ⚫ ɜ⚫

I liked Carter very much. He was quite pleasant, downright fun. He was intrigued by everything to do with his treatment. As a future scientist, he had to know all the technical points. He made me draw a schema of all the metabolic pathways, showing him the mechanism of action of every drug he would receive. He would study my charts for hours and then propose a new type of chemotherapy that might work better.

As independent as teenagers are, they treasure the comfort of a mother's hand or hug. They are rarely too proud in such circumstances to relinquish their hard-won control. Carter would have done the same. His mother rarely came into the treatment room while he was having a painful test or treatment. Tamara would not touch him.

Once he cried for her, and she fled the room. I held him in my arms as he wept silently for half an hour. When his tears were spent, he thanked me and left with Tamara. They walked down the hallway together without a word.

I must admit that I did not spend as much time with Carter as with my other patients. I struggled to treat this family in a nonjudgmental fashion but found it at times overwhelmingly difficult. I could not steel myself to spend anymore time with them than was absolutely necessary. Carter sensed that, I think, and for that I've always had regret.

There was something in his mother's attitude that I could not understand. She seemed unable to affirm him as other mothers cherish their cancer-afflicted children. I wanted Carter to cry out, *Deliver me from this woman!* But of course, he didn't. He was her son, and he loved her dearly.

One day a minor surgical procedure caused him a great deal of pain. Carter cried for his mother. She raged at him and told him to act like a man. But she called him "Robbie," then left the room. I asked Carter, "Is 'Robbie' your middle name?"

"No. Robbie was my uncle. I never met him. He died before I was born."

The foreboding I had about this family would not go away. It was not for many years, long after Carter died, that I learned Tamara's story.

❧   ❧   ❧

Tammy was a beautiful child, sired by a distant father. She was the only girl in the family, the youngest child. As a three-year-old, she passed long hours standing before her mirrored closet, choosing her dress for the day. She longed for her father to notice her.

It was her oldest brother who paid her the most attention. He became her hero, played with her when the others told the little kid to take off. He liked war games, tommy guns, and such. On his wall was a poster of Attila the Hun. When Tammy got into fights, it was Robbie who fought her battles. She loved to come to his room to play.

She was six and he was fourteen when it started, one of those times she came to his room. No one else was home. She was pleased when he drew her close and set her on his lap. He rocked her and closed his eyes, rubbing her against him.

The first time he took her hand and asked her to touch him, she drew away. That's where boys were different from girls, what Mommy called their private parts. "It's okay, Tammy," he said, taking her hand again. "Don't I take care of you? I wouldn't do anything to hurt you. It will just be our secret. If you want to come to my room and play, then we will have our little secret."

The child loved her brother more than anyone in the world. The thought that he might not play with her was more than she could bear. And so she touched him where he asked. He held her hand, showed her how to please him. She was frightened when he groaned and seemed to be in another world. She tried to let go, but he held her hand tightly and kissed her.

That first night she had a nightmare and cried out in her sleep. As her mother came to comfort her, she found Robbie already in the hallway. "That's okay, Mom. I'll take care of her. I'll stay with her until she falls back asleep." And so, he held her and rocked her, and she was glad that he was there.

These trysts continued for three years. It was their secret, and he never hurt her, just showed her how to make him happy. And yet, the child had a sense of guilt and abandonment. Sometimes she wished that her parents would find out so that it would end. She felt dirty, yet she loved Robbie so much that she could not say no when he asked her to touch him in that special way.

It ended one night when Robbie came to her room. Their mother heard noise and went to check on Tammy. She screamed out and was quickly joined by her husband who throttled the boy, then slapped him hard in the face. Tammy pleaded for them not to hurt him, that it was her fault, not his. Robbie ran out of the house, grabbing the car keys on the way. His father screamed after him, "You're not my son. I disown you, you little piece of filth!"

ह्र   ह्र   ह्र

The police did not identify Robbie until the next morning. Two patrol cars pursued him in a high-speed chase after they saw him driving one hundred-twenty miles an hour down the highway.

The car caught fire as soon as it hit the telephone pole. They had to wait for the wreckage to cool before they could check the motor number against vehicle records. No identification was found on the body or in the car. The police considered it fortunate that it was a single-car accident, that no one but the driver was killed.

There was no service for Robbie, no obituary in the newspaper. The small-town headlines had already said more than enough. The parents explained to friends that the body was burned beyond recognition. It was simpler to have a private graveside service. They just set him in the ground without a marker.

Tammy was not there to see her brother committed to the earth. She was sobbing in her room, blaming herself for her brother's death. If she had not touched him, Robbie would never have died.

When her son was three years old, Tamara first noticed that Carter looked like her brother. By the time he was six years old, she found the likeness intolerable. From that time on, she never touched her son. That is, until the week of his death.

I suppose it was inevitable that Carter never did well. He faced death less than a year after his tumor was first discovered. To help with his pain, to try for another remission, we gave Carter more powerful chemotherapy. His pain was controlled, but an infection developed that caused his fever to climb.

Two teary-eyed nurses tried to restrain the boy onto a cooling blanket as his temperature and his body soared. They held his outstretched arms as I heard him cry out, "Oh God, tell me if you exist." Seven lasting words.

Can a woman forget her nursing child, or show no compassion for the child of her womb? Somehow, there had to be an answer for this almost motherless child's needs. If there was a God, surely he would reach out in mercy to this young man.

≀▲   ≀▲   ≀▲

I never knew what brought the change in Tamara and most likely never will. It was simply that all of a sudden she seemed to be freed to meet her son's needs. She took Carter home.

I visited them as often as possible. Although his body was deteriorating, the boy was at peace. I sat on his bed one day, still holding his hand after I finished checking his pulse, extending a medical touch into a more human one.

From his bed we could see some ducks climbing out of a pond and padding up onto a tennis court. Two neighbor boys were volleying with more vigor than skill that day. There was longing in Carter's eyes, a tiny benign spark of envy. But then he closed his eyes as if to blink them away and himself back to this room.

Carter thought that his temperature was going up again, and he was right. Tamara came quietly into the room, laid her hand on his forehead, confirmed his suspicion. Then she took a cool cloth and wiped her son's face. I moved away from the bed to see what would happen next.

She took a basin of water and a cloth, began to wash his body, then spread baby oil on his shoulders. The muscles relaxed, the body did not arch. Carter fell asleep, gently holding his mother's hand to his lips.

Her own lips met her son's hand gently before releasing it.

Tamara walked with me to my car. I could think of nothing to say. There was not much to discuss, medically speaking. All my unanswered questions were far too personal to pursue. I took my questions home with me, leaving Carter in his own bed, with his own family.

On the way back to the hospital, I remembered Carter's prayer to the God in whom his mother did not believe and an ancient promise as well: *Even if a mother were to forget, yet I will not forget you. Perhaps,* I thought, *there is a God who hears the prayers of the poor and afflicted. If there is a Creator of this universe, surely he must be generous enough to tell one dying boy, "Yes, I exist. And I love you."*

↜ ↜ ↜

After Carter's death, at home, there was a notice in the local newspaper. A memorial service would take place by the duck pond he could see from his window. Carter deserved to be honored and remembered, it said. He was Tamara Lowell's beloved son.

4

Hannah's Exultation

They brought the child to Eli. And Hannah said, "Oh, my lord! I am the woman who was standing here in your presence, praying to the LORD. For this child I prayed; and the LORD granted me the petition that I made to him. Therefore I have leant him to the LORD; as long as he lives—he is given to the LORD."

1 Samuel 1, 2

*S*he sat quietly in the waiting room reading *Family Circle*. Farm fresh, Hannah wore no makeup. Her sun-streaked hair was plaited into a single French braid. Until she looked up, there was nothing remarkable to note. But she did look up, filling the room with light as you beheld her eyes—striking green. Hannah looked back down at her magazine and blended back into the shadows.

She sat in the waiting area, dressed in blouse and jeans, no different from other mothers in the room. Yet I realized that that was exactly what distinguished her the most. Where was the freshly pressed dress or tasteful suit? Blue jeans are for later, battle fatigues for vets. Sammy was a new patient, but his mother dressed like an old-timer.

This was my image of Hannah when we first met and every time thereafter. If she was anxious about our first visit, I couldn't tell it from her face or clothes. As circumstances changed, Hannah integrated without compromising, accommodated without conceding. When I walked into the waiting area to call them,

Sammy was playing on the
lowed her five-year-old son
neither hovered over him r
arms.

Like his mother, the chil
yet, I knew that their pediatrici
worst fears. There was a lump
growing rapidly in Sammy's nec
talized nearer to home for man
antibiotics. Now it was time for ᵤ see a cancer
specialist for children. Hannah knew why she was
there. And so did Sammy.

I've seen her face and his in my imagination so often that time does not seem to diminish the clarity of
the picture. There was something about the triad we
formed—Hannah, Sammy, and I—that drew us together those many years ago. It is not an easy thing to
define.

Long ago, we put aside a distance that was never
meant to be. Hannah and I were closer than sisters. We
were like mother and mother to the same child. It was
a mark of her deep trust that she was willing to share
her son with me. Sammy helped close the distance the
first day.

When I walked with them to an examining room,
he looked up at me shyly. Sammy ran his hand through
his freshly punked hair and sighed, and with the sigh,
sucked in on his cheeks, deepening his dimples. There
were flecks of gold in the green that sparkled when the
light hit his irises, flickered from his eyes to mine and

mond earring in his left earlobe. Finally, a little boy's titter, and Hannah prodded ell, aren't you gonna ask her?"

"Ask me what?" I was intrigued by the family secret, the covert glance that leaped and rebounded from boy to mom to boy. *Whatever it was must be worth knowing,* I thought.

Sammy cupped his mouth to my ear, whispered moistly into it, "Can I have your autograph?" I stood bolt upright, startled by his question.

"My autograph? Nobody's ever asked me for my autograph before! I am so honored."

"Patty said you're real famous." Hannah quickly explained that Patty was his favorite nurse. She was the one who stayed with him in the Intensive Care Unit when he was most frightened. Just one week earlier, Sammy was discharged from that hospital and now was coming to another. He was afraid to come to a big hospital, and his nurse had calmed his fears in the best way she could imagine.

"You're going to see *Dr. Komp*?" she asked him. "Why, she's so famous!" Sammy was impressed. Next to his mother, Patty was the most important woman in the world. And now, I seemed fortunate enough to be joining that short list of feminine luminaries.

I fetched a reprint of an article I had published and signed it for Patty. Then I gave Sammy a publicity photograph that I found in my desk, and I autographed it regally. He was smitten.

The child went to the lab for his blood work with the photo pressed to his chest. He showed it to each technician he could find. They all told him that I had never given any of them an autographed photo. He blushed with pleasure. I was blushing, too. The blood-flush in our cheeks, Sammy's and mine, sealed our kinship.

❧   ❧   ❧

Sammy never really responded well to treatment. Nothing we could offer would eradicate the errant clone of cancer that defied the best we had. After our first meeting, there were few days that he was in his own home. We tried to send him out on pass a few times so that he could visit his puppy and sleep in his own bed.

Each day, Hannah saw me walk softly into another child's room, suspecting the reason for my uncharacteristic solemnity. Every week, she read other mothers' tears, sensed the parting of their sons and daughters. There were no secrets on a children's ward. Wordlessly, mysteries were shared.

She played music for Sammy, there in the hospital. One day he heard these words: *Our God is an awesome God. He reigns in heaven above in wisdom and power and love.* The words enkindled his imagination.

"You're kidding, Mom!" he said. "God is awesome?"

Hannah thought about it, then answered with great confidence, "Sure!"

"God is *awesome*?" he repeated. "Does God wear an earring?"

"Well," thought Hannah, "he would if he wanted to!"

"Awesome!" was her little one's response.

≥● ≥● ≥●

I watched Hannah watch us. Many a time when we made rounds, she stood close, listening carefully to our medical chatter. She appeared more a part of our team than an outsider to the medical mystery. This was her son, after all. Hannah was not to be shut out.

During his illness, the disease filled Sammy's brain. First it robbed him of his speech, next of his vision, finally of his ability to walk. Never have I felt as frustrated as when that tumor progressed, robbing Sammy of everything that we prize about being human. And yet, Sammy maintained a serenity that was beyond explanation. He could barely move but did what he could without complaint. He could finger his little yellow tape recorder and play his awesome tape.

He was in a room with three other brain-damaged boys, worse off than he, if such was possible. One child had fallen out of a fourth-story window. Another had been beaten. The third was the hapless victim of a hit-and-run driver. The room was a vegetable garden, filled with wilting young life. Mothers sat patiently at their sides, encouraging their sons with their therapy, hoping and praying for a miracle.

The dimples in his steroid-plumped cheeks were flattened out, altering his smile. Sammy used the little strength he had in his right hand to operate his tape recorder. Hannah and I chatted on, discussing his latest test results. From time to time, we would look over to Sammy. He had lain back and listened to his music with the volume turned down so as not to disturb others in the room.

As we spoke, we heard a blast of song: *We declare that the kingdom of God is here! The blind see, the deaf hear, the lame man is walking. Sicknesses flee at his voice. The dead live again and the poor hear the good news. Jesus is King, so rejoice!* We were startled, as were the others in the room but we all heard the words.

Without being asked, Sammy turned down the volume when that song was finished. He continued to listen quietly to the other songs. Then, with the little strength that he had in the tips of his fingers, he rewound the tape. He played it quietly until he reached the same song.

We declare that the kingdom of God is here ... Again, the blind, the deaf, and the lame in that room were startled to attention. It was obvious that Sammy knew what he was doing. I went to the side of his bed and took his hand. He smiled his sunny smile.

"You really believe that, don't you, kiddo?" I asked. And he nodded vigorously. Sammy believed. But did I? In his childlike faith, this six-year-old found comfort in these words. No, *more than comfort*. He seemed to find peace and meaning for his life. But his apparent peace brought anxious thoughts into my own mind.

What would Sammy think of his awesome God if he was not healed? Surely the prophet meant spiritual blindness, not physical. Then I realized that the fears were mine and mine alone. *Truly I tell you, unless you change and become like children, you will never enter the kingdom of heaven.* It was my God who was too small. Sammy and his awesome God shared the secret of his peaceable kingdom.

ॐ   ॐ   ॐ

The child was transferred to the Intensive Care Unit and kept my beeper ringing busily when I was at home. While he was in the hospital, there were very few quiet evenings.

It was such a day one Sunday when I took out a few hours to teach my junior-high-school Sunday school class. Thirty-two rascals kept my focus on life, and I used my guitar like a mighty weapon. As long as I could keep them singing, I was in control and we were all happy. Then my beeper went off. I left the class for a few minutes to use the phone in the pastor's study. When I returned, they sat there silently, waiting for me to say something.

What could I say? What could they or should they understand about a child younger than they, clinging to life on a respirator? I felt their eyes on me as I sat down. The children anticipated that I might need prodding, so they had elected a representative, a doctor's daughter. "Did somebody die?" she asked.

Fool that I was, I did not even realize that the children knew what type of doctor I was. Did healthy pubescents even know what it meant to be a "pediatric oncologist"? My innocence and theirs were lost that day together. As carefully as I could, I told them about Sammy. They continued to stare and wait. It was clear that they were looking for more than a story. So I suggested that we pray for Sammy, together.

After church, I went to the hospital and spoke with Hannah. I told her about the children, how they had challenged me, how we had prayed together, how I had again learned to never, never again underestimate a child.

Several days later, Sammy died. I stood at his bedside, silent and saddened. Hannah handed me a letter. It was for my Sunday school class. In it, she thanked the children for their prayers and told them that God had indeed answered their prayers. *The dead live again. Jesus is King, so rejoice!* Sammy was with his awesome God.

❧   ❧   ❧

I've thought about our first meeting often. Long after I knew Hannah well, I kept replaying that waiting room scene, imagining what she was thinking as she waited for me to call out Sammy's name.

I recalled her face at Sammy's bedside in the ICU as I primed myself to deliver the latest grim news. But she was at peace. Each visit, she smiled at me gently and inquired, "How are you this morning?" This woman was a gift.

She looked just the same that day at his funeral, except for the dark dress and the tears that filled her eyes when she saw me. I walked to the chapel, weeping myself. And yet, as we embraced, it was not for herself alone that she wept. She wept for me as well.

"Oh, Diane, I'm so sorry. You lose so many children. I wanted to give you one child who would live. I wanted Sammy's life to be a gift to you."

As long as I had known her, I still was stupefied. What type of woman was this who could lose her son and grieve for the loss that another woman might feel for the same child?

In some sense, Sammy was never fully Hannah's, simply hers on loan. How could this young mother fathom what it was like for me, a middle-aged childless woman, to "mother" other women's children and lose so many? I hardly knew, myself, and yet she seemed to know.

&. &. &.

Hannah visited the hospital often after Sammy's death. The bonds that tied us were too strong for death to sever. Often, one or more of her younger children came along. Hannah never shut them out of this part of her life while Sammy lived, and she would not exclude them now.

Little Amy seemed particularly pleased to come back each time, as if she were in a place where Sammy still lived. As young as she was, she thought of us as people who loved and cared for her brother. Our "home" was a safe place where she could freely speak of Sammy.

These visits always pleased me, bringing a welcome break to a day's drudgery. Although her son was gone, our journey together was not yet complete. After seeing Hannah, it was easier for me to face a newer mother. It was on one of these occasions, with Amy at her side, that she sought to speak to me privately.

"I've never told you this before. The day that Sammy died, he said something that told me that he knew that the end had come. He said, 'I want to go home.' The nurses thought he meant home to Lovingston, but I knew what he really meant. I knew that he knew that this earth was never his real home."

Years had passed since Sammy's death. You could no longer speculate that she was operating on the emotional high that often surges after a loss. She was so calm, so radiant. I had the sense of being on holy ground, speaking to someone who knew what it means to love her child with her whole heart but to love God more.

Hannah wasn't looking at me as she was speaking. Her gaze was on another time and place as she exulted, "I was there when he was born. I was there when he went home. It was such a privilege to be his mother. I am so blessed." And so was I.

5

Elena's Prayer

The daughter of Pharaoh came down to bathe at the river. She saw a basket among the reeds. When she opened it, she saw a child. He was crying, and she took pity on him.

Exodus 1, 2

*S*he sat in a cornfield, transfixed by the blue morning mist that enfolded the distant volcano. There were rumors that the *judiciales* had come, searching for guerrillas in the highlands of Guatemala. It was hard to believe that such a beautiful land could be so violent. Elena sighed and replaced her flat basket on her head before she headed home to the shack.

They caught her as soon as she entered the room. Her youngest sister was cowering in a corner, sobbing. Her eyes followed the child's animal-wild gaze. Their mother lay motionless on the floor, bloodied, naked, disemboweled. Elena spun around to see one of the *militares* drag her brother into the room. His eyes were swollen shut, his mouth filled with blood. There was a gun to his head, and he was sobbing.

The soldiers had raped their mother before they murdered her. Now it was Elena's turn. One of the *militares,* big-bellied, with rotten teeth and pig-sweating face, reached down to undo his trousers. In less than a bloody minute, he rolled off her, leaving her dress stained, reeking of his brief presence.

Elena lay there unmoving, afraid that he might start all over again. Instead, his *companeros* took his place, one after the other, all night. She tried to imagine herself far away from this pathetic village with its tin-roofed shanties, away from a land bent on annihilating its entire Indian population. A soldier slapped her so hard that her body went crashing into the *bajareque* wall and she lost consciousness. Her eyes stared up, vacantly; blood poured from her mouth. Despite their intentions, she survived. The next day she awoke to find her mother, father, three sisters, and two brothers dead and mutilated. All because her father was an *indio*.

Fearing that the soldiers would return, Elena fled with the little food she could find. They had stolen their few miserable chickens. She wrapped her provisions in her basket and herself with a shawl for protection from the night air as she crept deep into the highlands.

When her food ran out, she stole at night from village to village. It was a mark of the poverty in that region that there was so little garbage to be found. Very rarely, there was a slow-moving scrawny chicken to snatch. It was frightening at night, alone in the mountains, but she feared the animals less than the human predators who might find her hiding place. She kept on the move in the highlands to avoid being spotted by either the guerrillas or the federal troops.

ء‌ا   ء‌ا   ء‌ا

At first she didn't know what was happening to her body, why her breasts were budding out, her belly swelling. But then she knew.

Her first reaction was to be ashamed, to hate what was in her that the soldiers had left behind. And yet, the child was also hers, part Indian. She would not let them wipe her people off the face of the earth. Elena might perish, but she swore that her baby would survive. And once it was born, she would find a way for the child to have a better life.

She thought of the few prayers she had heard the rare times that a priest came as far as their little village. Elenita tried to remember what the angel said to Maria when she, young, yet unmarried, found herself pregnant. *The Lord is with you. Don't be afraid.* She struggled to recall Maria's response. *My soul magnifies the Lord, and my spirit rejoices in God my Savior.*

Every night, she fell asleep with those words on her lips and her *tzute* wrapped around her. She prayed that God would guard the baby that she carried. She wept for her murdered mother, mourned her loss. There was no one to explain to a young girl that which was happening to her body.

But what of Maria? Did she tell her own mother at first? How could she convince a pious family that she was pregnant by God? Her cousin Elizabeth believed the angel story that Maria told and shared her outrageous joy. That was what Elena prayed for—the gift of outrageous joy, the ability to bless her baby for the gift of its companionship. *God has looked with favor on the lowliness of his servant.*

ॐ   ॐ   ॐ

It was at dawn when the pains began. Elena rocked herself, hidden in another cornfield. She focused on the same distant volcano, allowing field and mist to midwife her. She dared not cry out lest she be found. As if to parrot her pangs, a bright orange glow erupted through the mist, crowning the volcano. With each pain, she remembered that other young woman who was far from home when her own time came. *The Lord is with me!* was Maria's exclamation. *Maria's Son Jesus, stay with me!* Elena prayed as a molten river snaked its way down the volcano, and her little daughter burst into the world.

She named the baby *Gabriella* after Maria's angelic visitor. She held the infant to her hunger-flattened breast and was amazed at the strength with which the baby sucked. The mother was wasting away, but the baby was fat. Elena might not survive, but the infant was sturdy and fighting for life.

There was no moon or stars that night to guide her as she left the *altiplano* for the city far below. She heard the treacherous racing waters in the deep ravine below as she descended from the highlands and made her way to the city.

She left the baby in the basket on the steps of a church, snugly wrapped in her shawl. Certain that the nuns would find it quickly, she stole back to the highlands, unprotected from the night air. *Maria's Son, Jesus, stay with my Gabriella,* she prayed as she collapsed to the ground. She had finished the task that had kept her alive all those months. There was a smile of incomparable joy on her lips as she surrendered to the chilling darkness.

ᨠ   ᨠ   ᨠ

It was the crying that woke Father Carrera. He stumbled out of his house next to the church and found a bright Indian cloth in motion. There was no one in sight—there rarely was when these babies were left. *These villages never seem to change,* he thought. *And there is no priest who will stay there and teach them a better way.*

The last missioner was killed by the military when he tried to organize the peasants. These young priests all seem to get radical when they work in the highlands. Better for a priest to stay here in the squalor of the city. Just last week two nuns were raped and murdered while the soldiers forced a young seminarian to look on. They left the young man for dead, but now he is safely on his way back to Iowa where corn can be grown in more peaceful circumstances.

The baby continued to cry, so he lifted the basket and headed for the convent. The sisters were dwindling in number, but they would care for this baby. They had contacts in El Norte who seemed to find families who wanted these babies. If not, there was always the orphanage, already teeming with the orphans of the *desaperecido,* the "disappeared." But this one was a squaller! She would wake the whole city before the first rooster had anything to say about today.

ॐ   ॐ   ॐ

Thousands of miles from the Guatemalan highlands, another mother was in labor. Tanya's husband was at her side for the birth of her first child. Sean would be there again with each pregnancy, holding her hand. Over the years they would be three times together in such a room. Only the first time did they take a baby home.

Their first child was named Elizabeth, a sunny Gerber baby sporting a wisp of blonde hair. She slept through the night from the second night on, this dream child. Then a year later, Christopher was born. He was a handsome boy-child with thick, black hair. But his liver and spleen were swollen, making him look painfully pregnant.

That was when I met Tanya and Sean for the first time. Just before Christopher died, we found a rare blood incompatibility. We knew that this condition would get worse with each child. There was no vaccine against this like the one available for "Rh babies." The young couple was distraught. How could a baby die so quickly?

But they were young and healthy and they still had Lizzy. Six months later, Tanya was pregnant again. This time, they stayed close to home, avoiding crowds and sick people. *Perhaps Tanya had caught some virus,* they thought, *and passed it on to the baby. Better to play it safe.*

Christopher's death had forewarned us, and for the next pregnancy the perinatal team was on standby. Everything went smoothly until the seventh month. My telephone rang when Tanya arrived in the OB suite. We tried to give the baby a blood transfusion while she was still in Tanya's womb, but labor started, and the mother was transferred to the Labor Room.

A nurse looked worried. After she saw the monitor, she left the room to call Dr. Kelly. Sean saw the moving, white line on the monitor and the digits flashing out above. He had seen enough of these machines to worry himself. His brow furrowed when he saw the number displaying the fetal heart rate. A baby's heart rate shouldn't be that slow. Tanya had another strong labor pain and gripped his hand. The baby's heart rate dropped even lower.

Dr. Kelly was in her blue scrubs when she came in. She, too, frowned when she saw the monitor. "Tanya, I think the safest thing to do is a Caesarean. That baby wants to come out as soon as possible, and I think we should help her."

Tanya nodded, and the nurse wheeled her toward the operating room. Sean squeezed her hand so tightly that it turned white. "Please, dear God, not again! It can't be. Not this early!"

Amanda, their third child, was born dead. Tanya and Sean could not believe it had happened again and might happen to future babies. How could this be? They were both healthy. They both wanted a large family. Why was this happening to them?

After Tanya was asleep in her hospital room, Sean went to his mother's home and took six-year-old Lizzy in his arms. "No baby, Daddy?" she asked. He didn't know what to say to his daughter. Tears filled his eyes. "Don't cry, Daddy," the child tried to console him. "It's okay. God will give us a baby. You'll see, Daddy. God has already made a baby for us to take care of."

૨૰   ૨૰   ૨૰

Tanya and Sean tried for years to adopt a baby. Their problem was that they had a living child. They would not be high up on an agency list. They called me once to ask me if I had any ideas, but I didn't. It was a frustrating time. But when they were sad, Lizzy would come and hold them close. "Don't cry. God has already made a baby for us. You'll see."

It was a friend who told them about special children who needed adoption. And soon they were talking to an agency about an older child, a seven-year-old girl, Lizzy's own age.

They came home to tell Lizzy and show her a picture. The child was as dark as their daughter was fair.

But when she saw the picture, Lizzy lit up. "That's our baby! That's my new sister that God had already made for us. She looks like an angel!"

᠊᠊᠊᠊᠊᠊᠊

They met Gabriella at the airport. She was accompanied by a nun from the convent orphanage. Gaby clung to the little woman shyly, amazed by all the new sights and sounds around her. It was Lizzy who went over to her first and put her arms around her.

"You're my sister. God sent you to us. We're going to take care of you. Everything is going to be all right. You'll see." She took the child's hand and led her over to Tanya and Sean who hardly knew what to do except follow Lizzy's lead. They stood there embracing the two girls, weeping. When they looked up, the nun was gone. All the child's possessions were in a small bag woven with an Indian design. They took her small hand and brought Gabriella home.

Lizzy insisted on sharing a room with her new sister so that she wouldn't be afraid in the dark. She showed her every corner of the house, not the least bit concerned that Gaby spoke no English. She picked out her favorite doll and gave it to her new sister, her first gift.

After dinner they found Gaby at the window, looking out and weeping. That night in bed, she sobbed. Lizzy crawled into bed with her and held her in her arms. "Don't cry, Gaby. We love you. God sent you to us. You'll see." Lizzy would rock the child until she fell asleep. In the morning, Tanya and Sean would find them in bed together, intertwined.

At times Lizzy could be overwhelming. She was determined to teach her new sister everything that she knew. And Lizzy was a very bright little girl. She took out the family photo album. "This is Grandma and Grandpa Rhodes. You'll meet them at Christmas. Did you ever meet your grandparents? Do you even know who your mother was?" The chatter was constant. Although Tanya didn't think that Gaby understood a word, she was reassured by Lizzy's confidence about their new life together.

Every night, after supper, they would find Gaby by the window with tears in her eyes. And every night she would cry in her bed until Lizzy came and stilled her fears. Tanya and Sean started to worry. Most of all, they worried whether Lizzy was taking on too much responsibility for a seven-year-old child.

Tanya called to ask if I could check Gaby out for medical problems. There were none to be found. I suggested contacting the orphanage of the Little Sisters of Jesus, where she had grown up, to ask if there was anything that the sisters recognized. The Mother Superior told them about the circumstances of the child's arrival.

Gaby was found on their doorstep, crying, and cried almost constantly for the next three months until a new sister came to their order. The only way the infant would sleep was to be rocked by Sister Maria, the nun who accompanied her on the flight to the United States. She could pacify the infant when no one or nothing else could.

When she was older, the child would sneak to the sister's room whenever she had night terrors, and they would find them in bed together in the morning. And yet it was Sister Maria who insisted that they must find a real home for her, that she should not grow up in an orphanage.

At Christmastime, Lizzy insisted that they dress alike. Lizzy carefully placed the photo of them, smiling together, in the album next to the pictures of the babies who no longer were alive, next to her own pictures as an only child. "God did not mean for me to be an only child," she would explain to Gaby. "Mommy and Daddy have so much love that it just wouldn't be fair. So God brought you to us so that you could be in our family album and we could love you."

The two girls would walk to school hand in hand and sit next to each other in the classroom. With Lizzy for a tutor, Gaby's English was coming along rapidly. Tanya and Sean decided to try separate rooms for the girls but abandoned that plan after three sleepless, sobbing nights. They asked Lizzy to try to sleep in her own bed, to help Gaby get used to sleeping alone.

One day, while cleaning, Tanya took out Gaby's Indian sack that came with her from the orphanage. In it she found a dog-eared photo of the nun, Sister Maria. She bought a small silver frame for it in a shop that day and placed it on Gaby's bedside table. When the child saw it that evening, she tore it out of the frame and held it to her, rocking and weeping. It was then that Tanya decided what she needed to do. She called the convent.

"Mother Superior," she began, "I know that this is a very unusual request. But I know that you want what is best for Gaby. She's still having problems adapting, and I think it would be a tremendous help if Sister Maria could come here and live with us for a while. I don't know what that will mean for her vows, but if there's a way, we promise that we'll help her however possible."

"You're right, Señora Rhodes, that is a most unusual request. Sister Maria is a most devout member of our order. She prays for all the unwanted and orphaned children of these villages. She devotes herself to the memory of the Holy Innocents."

"What's her story?" Tanya asked. "Do you know anything about the woman?"

"She's never told us, my child, and we have never asked. You must understand the sadness of the poor people who come to us. Forgive me for my impatience. These are trying times. We are here to be her family now. You are asking for her to leave her family."

"I just know that it's important to Gaby. Somehow I know your Sister Maria can help this one child even more than her prayers help all the other children. Can you trust a mother's heart? Do you understand what I'm trying to say?"

"I can only promise to pray about it. And ask the other sisters. That is all I can promise," came the answer.

"We'll be praying, too," said Tanya. "Please tell Sister Maria that we pray for her every day."

"Please pray for all of us," she murmured. Tanya heard exhaustion in the woman's voice. "These are difficult times for the peasants here. And when we try to help them, we ourselves must be ready to suffer and die."

❧ ❧ ❧

It was Lizzy who decided that they should decorate the whole house to welcome Sister Maria. She went with Tanya to pick out curtains and a bedspread for the room where she would sleep. Lizzy insisted that she feel at home with them. Then Lizzy took Gaby's hand and led her over to the party favors to buy special balloons. Tanya had never seen Gaby so excited.

Tanya was sure they had made the right decision. And for Mother Superior, it evolved as an answer to prayer. Two more lay cathechists in the region had been murdered by the death squads. The *militares* announced that the sisters must vacate the convent. It would become a command post for the federal troops.

Sister Maria would be assigned to the Rhodes as Gaby's nanny. She would continue with her prayers while the child was in school. In her heart, Mother Superior wished that Gaby and Sister Maria weren't the only ones to find a compassionate solution. She would bring the nun with her when she returned, defeated, to her order's mother house in New England.

At home, the children insisted on decorating the room themselves. Lizzy and Gaby blew up all the balloons and hung festive banners. Tanya was glad they had something to keep them out of mischief while she planned the welcome dinner. In three hours, Sister Maria would be at the Bradley Airport. Lizzy and Gaby closed the door behind them when they finished the room, wanting it to be a surprise. Tanya smiled.

The scene at the airport was what Tanya and Sean expected. The child ran to the nun and wouldn't let go of her. They kept hugging and weeping, happily reunited. Gaby chattered away, hardly letting Sister Maria get a word in. She introduced the nun to Lizzy. Those were the only words Tanya and Sean understood. My sister, Lizzy.

Sister Maria was overwhelmed by their house. Their modest raised ranch seemed like a luxury villa to her. From the nun's face, Tanya knew that this was the right decision. She hoped that her order would let Sister Maria stay for a very long time. The children took her by the hand to show her to her room.

With great fanfare, the girls opened the door. The room was filled with balloons. Festooned across the wall over the bed was a large banner: WELCOME HOME, NITA.

"Lizzy," Tanya said. "Her name is Maria, not Nita."

"No, Mommy," answered the child. "Sister Maria is her religious name. Her real name is Elena. Her family always called her Elenita, little Elena. Gaby calls her Nita . . ."

6

Hagar's Flight

*And God heard the voice of Ish-
mael; and the angel of God called to
Hagar from heaven, and said to her,
"What troubles you, Hagar? Do not
be afraid; for God has heard the
voice of the boy where he is. Come,
lift up the boy and hold him fast
with your hand, for I will make a
great nation of him."*

Genesis 16, 21

*I*t was in a little grocery store run by a man from her uncle's village that Hagar first saw him. She was sent by her mother to buy red lentils, goat cheese, and fresh, flat Turkish bread. He came in the crowded little shop in the Kreuzberg section of Berlin with another man. He was a "guest worker" as they called them. Newly arrived in Germany, he intended to make his fortune in this wealthy Western land.

He was taller than the other men Hagar knew, her father's friends. His eyes were a brighter brown and very direct. When he looked at her, she looked down modestly. Hagar wouldn't want him to guess her thoughts. But then, she really did.

The next time she saw him, he was in a café drinking thick Turkish coffee with three other men. The men were smoking and laughing when she spotted him. She kept her eyes down but noted that he saw her pass. His glance followed her all the way home. Hagar smiled secretly.

That evening, while the others slept, Hagar lay awake thinking about her future. Life in Ankara had been difficult. There was no work for her father there. True, the outskirts of Ankara were better than the small village where her cousins lived. But to Hagar, Berlin was pure luxury. She had seen how the Germans lived. Her mother worked as a maid for such a family. They were very polite with their maid but somewhat distant, to Hagar's way of thinking. At least, they were honest and fair.

Hagar learned a little of their language—more than her mother—from the children of this house. She looked around her family's tiny room and then thought about the grand flat in which her mother's employers lived. It seemed that these Germans worked hard, and that was how these possessions came to them. If she could only find a man who was a hard worker, someday she might live in luxury as well.

૱ ૱ ૱

His name was Ibrahim. She heard his friend address him as she walked behind them on the street one day. She kept a slight distance so that he would not know she was there with her little brother. She wanted to learn everything she could about him.

He spoke with his friend of a new opportunity and high wages. There was a contractor looking for men newly arrived from Turkey. They would be rich within a short time. As she came close to her apartment building, she motioned to little Mustafah to run ahead. Then she ran after her brother, passing the men, yelling at the child in rapid-fire Turkish. She saw Ibrahim turn and note her entering the building. As she closed the door, she looked directly at him, and he nodded his respect.

It was the same evening that he came to talk with her father. The two men went to the local café and the nuptial negotiations began.

🐦   🐦   🐦

Her mother's employer found a job for the new bride with another family. Hagar was proud that she could contribute to their meager income. Her husband took all their earnings to send home to his impoverished family. Still, she hoped that one day they, too, would have a fine apartment.

It was springtime when her clothes fit too tightly. Her mother laughed, "Pray that Allah will send you a son. Then all will go well with your husband." So she did.

Ismael came into the world with a lusty scream that satisfied the midwife. Hagar was happy that she had given her husband a healthy son. Ibrahim was pleased with his son and tender with him and Hagar. But he spoke of returning to Turkey, to that tiny village far from the city life of Ankara.

Hagar was stunned with the news. From the moment her family arrived in Germany, she had never thought to return to the poverty she had known in Turkey. She stood on the train platform, a study in brown and gray. A two-tone kerchief covered her hair.

The buttons of her mud-brown sweater strained to protect her from the cold. She gathered a plain gray coat around her to shield her from the wind that blew across her pregnant body.

What did wealth mean in a tiny village where Islamic custom supplanted federal regulations in everyday life? In Germany she had far more freedom than she had ever known before. What could she look forward to there? Hopefully, her second child would also be a boy. The father laughed and played with his son as Hagar watched her life pass from west to east.

૨ૐ ૨ૐ ૨ૐ

Life was very difficult for Hagar in this village. Ibrahim's relatives treated her like a foreigner and criticized her Western ways. She gave birth to their second child, a daughter. For the next few years, daughter followed daughter. As his father had before him, Ibrahim took a second wife. She bore him three sons in as many years.

Some ten years after their return, Ibrahim developed a cough that racked his body at night. Hagar begged him to see a German-trained doctor in Ankara and traveled with him on a crowded bus. It broke down en route to the city, and they huddled together during the night as the driver waited for dawn to start the repairs. When dawn came, Ibrahim was dead.

After his death, Ibrahim's mother treated her like a servant. Hagar longed for her own mother and the prospect of a future for her son. She thought of how the German family had treated her. And at least they had paid her money for her menial work. So she and her children started back on the road to Ankara and from there to Germany. From these two hostile worlds, Hagar chose the lesser of the two evils.

ह   ह   ह

Ten years later, Hagar's mother still spoke little German. Hagar scolded her mother, warned her that her own life would be better if she looked out for herself better. But her mother lashed back. Her daughter was a foreigner to her own people. And with so many fancy ideas! Who was the daughter to advise the mother? Life was not meant to be exciting, Hagar. We are only meant to survive.

She worked hard now to learn more German. Hagar determined that through education her children would find their way out of a ghetto existence and take their place among doctors, lawyers, and other learned ones.

They were back in Berlin for only two weeks when Ismael took ill. She fought the sense of panic rising biliously from the pit of her stomach. This could not be happening to her twice! He was her son, her sun, her hope. She meant for Ismael to grow up, to become a doctor, to make his way between the two worlds. It could not be happening to him. It was through Ismael that she would be vindicated.

It was a week later that she found herself with him in a doctor's office at the medical school. There, she read eyebrows instead of reports. Words can evade, even lie. Even if only briefly, the eyes must tell the truth. The nurses were gentle with her and treated her with respect, but the doctors confused her with too many words. In her head and heart, a voice screamed obscenities that drowned them out.

∂⃛ ∂⃛ ∂⃛

I met Hagar the morning after Ismael was admitted to the hospital. I was on sabbatical that year, visiting a children's cancer ward and my German counterparts. There seemed to be many Turkish children in this most Western of European countries.

"I think we pediatricians are the only ones in Germany who love the Turks," suggested one pediatrician. There was a touch of romantic hyperbole in his words. But if it was an overstatement, it couldn't have been very far from the truth. In my mailbox that morning I had found a neo-Nazi flyer: AUSLÄNDER STOP. Stop admitting foreigners. Don't let them assimilate, it said. Because they "respected" their culture and religion, this group wanted to see them sent back where they could be fully appreciated.

"Many of our own young people are too pessimistic to become parents," my colleague continued. "Our own birthrate is dropping. We have something to learn from the Turks, what it means to have a heart for children and the courage to continue to bring them into this dangerous world."

ﻬﻬ ﻬﻬ ﻬﻬ

Hagar sat between us and her son as we entered the room to make rounds. She was polite and respectful, as was the boy. He was a bright-eyed lad with golden brown eyes that danced. There was hope in those eyes. Ismael knew that he was sick, but he had faith in the German medicine that he would one day study. He believed that we could make him well. His German was limited, but there was promise in his eyes that he would quickly learn.

The tests were all in, and the results clear. Ismael had leukemia, but the sort that holds promise for cure. The treatments in Germany were so successful that American cancer centers were trying them. I was with one of the German oncologists when he went back to the room to talk to Hagar. There were many side effects to the treatment that required explanation.

I watched Hagar as the doctor explained, satisfied that she understood all he said. A foreigner myself, I knew all the alien's tricks. Her German seemed quite adequate. What she lacked in formal education, she more than compensated for with common sense. This was no woman to underestimate.

There was no hospital staff member available who was fluent in Turkish. It fell to Hagar to translate for her son. My colleague worried that she might hold details back, not impart all that he had said. The oncologist pleaded with her to translate it all: The disease was serious, that he might die. The treatment was serious, what he must suffer if he was not to die. And yet, I could see from the look on the child's face that Ismael had heard only good news, not the bad.

The doctor asked again, "Please be sure to tell him everything. Leave nothing out."

She looked at him defiantly. "I've told him all. There is nothing left to say."

I cannot describe Hagar better to you, the emotions that she felt, the pain she confronted. There was a distance, uncommon even in Germany, that she did not wish to bridge. Most of the other mothers on this ward were curious about me, the American anomaly. Not Hagar. Her longings had nothing to do with me. It was as if the kerchief that concealed her hair shut me out from a closer view. Hagar remains for me an intimation, viewed in an antique mirror, dimly.

For the next three days, the chemotherapy was in full force. From morning to night, Ismael was sick. Hagar sat by his side, between us and him. But the days were not all tests and medicine. For a few hours each day, a school teacher came. German textbooks filled Ismael's bedside stand. He was a diligent student, and with his teacher he hunted for the words he sought.

Hagar took time away when the teacher came, the only hour away from his side. His mother was not there that third day of chemotherapy as we made our rounds. His teacher was there, Ismael's fond co-

conspirator. She spoke no Turkish, but she understood this bright young man. She stood back as we entered, *Halbgötter in weißen Kitteln*, the white-coated deities.

The youngster had studied us all, wordlessly understood the part that each of us played in this daily drama. Usually, when we made our rounds, Ismael looked first to the most senior doctor, the German professor, the one in charge, but it was my eyes he sought this time. His own eyes were no longer bright and dancing but those of a caged animal. For three days, without warning, he had vomited. It was to a fellow alien that he turned when he begged, "Bitte, nicht mehr." *Please, no more. Have mercy on me and stop all this sickness that I don't understand.*

&. &. &.

I was only a visitor there. I never heard the end of Ismael's story, nor Hagar's, but I think about them often. I think of Ismael, choose to believe that he survived, as have so many other children treated in that fine hospital. I think what it must have been like for him to face the chemotherapy without warning. I see his haunted eyes when, back home in America, I meet my newest patient. I slow down in my own explanations these days, take care to clearly communicate.

Ismael would be eighteen years old now, preparing for medical school if he followed his original dream. I imagine his choosing oncology for a career.

He seemed so bright and would have so much to offer his patients.

But most of all I think of Hagar, trapped between two cultures, valued by neither. No one at the hospital bore her ill for the way she shielded her son. She did her best even if it was different from our way. No one loved Ismael more than she; no one could have done better. But the foreignness remained.

I thought about them much this year, seven years later. For me, it's another sabbatical year. For Germany, it is the year of Mölln, Rostock, and Solingen: Neo-Nazi gangs, arsonist attacks, and Turkish families burned to death. These extremists may number but a few, but their impact has been devastating. *Can it happen here again?*

Where I lived, hundreds of refugees continued to pour into Germany from every war-torn country in the world. Every week, you noted their increasing numbers on the streets. *Would it happen here again?* In a bookstore window, I saw a poster framed by a rainbow, a whisper of hope lettered in a modern German hand:

> *When an alien resides with you in your land, you shall not oppress the alien. The alien who resides with you shall be to you as a citizen among you. You shall love the alien as yourself.*

> Leviticus 19:33, 34

This ancient mandate from the eternal Law, lost to many in so-called "Christian lands," had been found by a faithful remnant. *The counsel of the LORD stands forever,* I thought, *the thoughts of his heart to all generations. Hagar, the LORD has heard you in your affliction.*

❧   ❧   ❧

I thought I saw her once in Berlin this year. It was only for a brief moment in a shop on Kurfürstendamm. The woman was smartly dressed, an elegant brown-and-gray scarf accenting a stylish camel coat. She was laughing with a young Turkish man. I could not be certain that it was Hagar and doubted that she would remember me. Was that Ismael with her?

Too late I turned, wanting so to know what had become of them both. But they were gone, and I was left there on Berlin's most fashionable boulevard to imagine what happened to them as aliens in this foreign land.

7

Rahab's Crimson Cord

Then Rahab let Joshua and the spies down by a crimson cord through the window, for her house was on the outer side of the Jericho city wall and she resided within the wall itself. Rahab the prostitute, with her family and all who belonged to her, Joshua spared. Her family has lived in Israel ever since.

Joshua 2, 6

*R*ahab lived and worked on the streets from the age of sixteen on. There was a fellowship she found there with other whores. They looked out for each other when no one else would. They were sisters who did not turn their heads away when she walked by.

There were days when she looked like a mannequin on the cover of *Ebony*. When Rahab was feeling well, her skin glowed like a glistening caramel crust, her eyes were fire-bright. But there were those other days—the days that crack seemed to overrule and overwhelm—when people like me might have crossed over to the other side of the street.

Three weeks after she gave birth to the child, Rahab left the baby with a friend. That was how LaVonne became a mother. Rahab was on her way out of town with a guy named Jo Jo. LaVonne suspected that the police were on their trail, the pimp's drug deals about to bust.

Rahab gave her child to a woman who had failed every alcohol rehab program in New Haven County.

LaVonne could drink past Antabuse, vomit her guts out, and then keep drinking. One time she kicked a policeman in the butt. He charged her with drunken disorderly conduct, yet he came to the drunk tank and pleaded with her.

"You're a fine woman, LaVonne," he argued with her. "You don't need this muck. You could make something of yourself. You could be a somebody. Hell, you are a somebody. Why don't you get sober?" Even Sergeant O'Connor (who attended AA faithfully himself) finally concluded that LaVonne was hopeless. LaVonne didn't see herself as much different from Rahab. She just had bigger dreams. Sometimes she went to church and sat in a back pew. Those good Christian folks never really looked her square in the eye when she was drunk.

The baby was a tiny thing, nameless as yet. The birth certificate simply read "Female Washington." LaVonne named her "Eva" after the mother of all living. The tiny child she held in her arms could mean a new beginning for them both. It was as if Rahab had thrown a lifeline to her friend. After Eva came into her life, LaVonne went to church regularly. No child of hers would be raised without the songs of her people. For the sake of her new daughter, LaVonne would try.

Long ago LaVonne sang in a gospel choir and would again if they let her. There was an emptiness in her belly that only found filling in God's house. Life had been hard as long as LaVonne remembered. Her people were like the children of Israel, wandering in time and space and ghetto. For LaVonne there had been one Egypt after another, but as long as she never forgot to sing, there would be hope. But she could not abide the preaching about sin.

Sometimes, LaVonne walked out right in the middle of the sermon. She listened to all the fine matrons murmur to each other under the brims of their flowered hats as she passed them by. They covered their mouths with their Bibles, as if she would not know that they were talking about her. But, with Eva, she tried again. She went to church with her baby and held her head high. She was sober in the sanctuary. There was nothing that folks could say about LaVonne when she went to church with her baby.

≈ ≈ ≈

Motherhood suited LaVonne well. She was up early every morning to bathe and feed her baby, read to her from books. LaVonne became a common sight in the Hill section of New Haven early mornings, strolling with her baby. By 10:00 A.M. they retreated back to the housing project before the drug dealers took over the street and the sound of Uzi fire could be heard. By midday you stayed away from windows and even below them.

LaVonne hadn't heard from Rahab since the day two years earlier that she had casually dropped the baby off. She had heard on the streets that she was in Niantic Women's Prison on a drug charge. Chances were that it was her pimp's sentence that his main lady was serving. Many of the prisoners had been coerced by their pimps or boyfriends to say that the dope was their own. The courts were more lenient with women. She would get out after a shorter sentence and escape a certain beating had she not agreed to take the fall for him. So much for the perks of Rahab's job.

The authorities were never consulted on this "adoption" nor did LaVonne seek welfare money to support the child. She simply took care of the child on her own. There was no way that they would have allowed her to keep the baby, had they known. They would do their own whispering, on paper.

Eva grew up a happy and friendly child whose mother adored but did not spoil her. To the staff in Primary Care, LaVonne was known as a reliable mother. No appointment was missed, no baby-shot delinquent. They had no reason to doubt that she was the baby's mother. LaVonne never asked for services that required the birth certificate to be produced. No one in the hospital seemed to notice as long as the baby was healthy.

It was one of the pediatric residents working in Primary Care Clinic who called me. She was worried about Eva because of persistent swollen glands in her neck. A two-week trial of potent antibiotics had not affected them in the least. The child's blood counts were not what they should be for a healthy child. These were all signs that pointed to a malignancy.

LaVonne watched me intently as I examined the child. Nothing fit. The pieces of the puzzle didn't seem to go together for me. I'm sure that I frowned. "You think it leukemia or somepin like that?" she asked. A very good question, since that was exactly what I was checking for.

"I have to tell you that it's a good possibility." I chose my words cautiously. "But none of the tests seems to confirm that. My recommendation is that we check some of that swollen gland under the microscope. It's called a biopsy. That's the next step."

"You gonna cut on ma chil'? I don' want nobody ta cut on ma baby! Ya hear?" And then she began to sob, pressing the child to her.

"It's okay," I tried to reassure her. "You can stay with Eva in the hospital. You can stay with her up to the time she goes into the operating room."

In my innocence, I did not realize the source of her concern. Once the child was in the hospital, once papers needed to be signed, once insurance needed to be checked, LaVonne's secret would be out. Her greatest fear was that the authorities would come and take away her baby.

I cannot say that the child-protection worker was pleased with the arrangement. But they were hard-pressed for foster homes, and the child was temporarily in our care. The biopsy of the lymph node didn't help in the least, and we were left with an enigma. As Eva remained in the hospital, we tried to solve two puzzles. One was her diagnosis. The other was her future. Neither one seemed easy to sort out. As she stayed under our care and test after test came back either negative or hard to interpret, the child's liver and spleen began to swell. Frustrated, I suggested another biopsy, this time the liver. Again, the results were non-specific. Twice I had to face LaVonne and tell her that we had taken risks but found no answers.

During this time, I noticed that there were two LaVonnes. There was the neatly dressed, bright, caring mother. But there was another LaVonne who missed appointments, especially when the child-protection worker was due. And she rarely stayed at night. The caseworkers seemed to expect only the second LaVonne. But I knew the other, the mother of this child, whose love for her seemed to be worth something.

❧   ❧   ❧

I suppose it was because the disease was still new that we didn't think of it at first. In fact, AIDS was reported in children for the first time while Eva was going through all the tests for the cancer that she did not have. AIDS was the "gay plague," someone else's problem. No one in the First World seemed to know that it belonged to women and children, too.

Eva was one of the first cases in our hospital. We barely knew what to do with her—or with each other. Was she contagious by simple touch? The infection-control team came once a week, and the rules changed as often.

Signs were hung. They never said that the patient had AIDS, just that there was a risk of "serious" infection. But by that time, most citizens of New Haven knew what type of patient got *Pneumocystis Carinii* pneumonia.

Fear came in with the signs. Ultimately, the signs were replaced by supply carts in the hallway by the door. But the dread of the plague did not leave with the plaques.

Something happened to LaVonne when we told her the news. The baby was born to another woman. She had no reason we knew of to fear for herself from the child. She sat looking down at the floor and said the words so quietly that I scarcely heard them. "I done call Nian'ic t'day ta check on 'er. Her mama, she daid."

There were no tears in her eyes, and yet I knew that she cared deeply for this woman. It was no small thing to take in a strange child. There must have been a bond between them.

"LaVonne, are you okay?" I asked. "She was your friend. It must hurt." The tears came.

"It done hurt a lot. She trusted me wit her baby. She be ma friend. She alway' took care a me when I done need takin' care of. Now she daid. Ma baby's mama daid."

She was crying when I came on Sunday afternoon to make rounds. And drunk. "They done kick me out o' church, them sweet life peoples. The elder, he say I go home 'n' sleep or somepin. They don' let me pray for ma baby's mama."

But the elder came that afternoon, prayed with her for Rahab and for her baby. He prayed for LaVonne, that she would follow Jesus and be healed of all her afflictions. LaVonne was there Monday night when I rounded before leaving for the evening. For the first time since the child was admitted, she stayed the whole night. I never saw her drunk again.

ᔥ ᔥ ᔥ

LaVonne and Eva had become part of our little landscape. According to the wisdom of the week, the child was to be confined to the room. All those who entered were to gown and glove and mask. As the weeks passed, we realized that we had more advances in rule making than we had in treatment. We didn't have any treatment. But at least for the present time, the child was stable.

We discharged her in LaVonne's care and saw her in the office for follow-up. But I saw LaVonne in the hospital more often than Eva came for outpatient visits. An increasing number of their little family of faith were under our hospital roof. LaVonne prayed with them, reading to them from the Bible.

Afternoons, Elder Edwards went from door-to-door on the Hill, a jean-clad simple man, defying the drug lords. He had aged considerably in the last year. It was just a year ago that his only son was taken from him, crossing from the school yard. The hit-and-run joyrider never stopped after he mowed the youngster down. The stolen car was found abandoned later that night.

The boy had been his father's hope, his heir to the ministry. Since early childhood, Terrance never once wavered in his faith. The young man was chosen by God, his father believed. It was the boy who gave the older man the energy to walk door-to-door. When he grew old, his son would be there, in his place. That had been his dream.

His son was gone to Jesus, but the work and the new plague went on. The preacher prayed the Lord of the harvest to send more laborers into the harvest. And the Lord sent Elder Edwards to the hospital to pray with a poor drunk whose friend had died of AIDS and whose little adopted daughter lay sick with the same illness. He prayed, and LaVonne believed. That was the last day she touched alcohol. LaVonne never looked back.

ॐ   ॐ   ॐ

For a year or so Eva seemed to do all right. Then she was admitted to the hospital for meningitis but quickly recovered. The child was still recovering in the hospital when it happened.

I was on my way to the Emergency Room one night to see a new patient when an ambulance nearly ran me down. They had barely parked when the back doors flew open and two EMTs jumped out with a stretcher. There was a blur of white sheets and black limbs, but staining it all, flowing like a mighty river, was a stream of blood.

On the stretcher was New Haven's latest sacrificial lamb. Hardened to the city's violence, I crossed over to the other side of the driveway and walked toward the pediatric section. Thank God, I did not have to care for adults!

I don't think I would have known until much later if the Edwardses hadn't driven up just then. Sister Edwards went with the stretcher as her husband ran to me. He was shaking so hard that I located two chairs where we could sit in the corridor. I took his hands, felt the jackhammer reverberation of his body in mine.

It was after prayer meeting that night, coming out of the church, that an innocent victim was caught in cross fire. You didn't even ask why people were shooting anymore. Even the children could tell you it started over drugs.

An anesthesiologist ran by us, joining the Code 12 team. There was an emergency page for a thoracic surgeon. The corridor was a commotion of blurred blue scrub suits, converging on LaVonne's stretcher.

"She was clean, Doc," he sobbed without tears. "She got herself sober. The Lord healed her of all the craving for booze. She was an inspiration to all the folks she visited."

For the longest time, I held his hand and felt his body convulse. The elder was a broken man. His wife came toward us from the direction they had taken LaVonne. There were tears in her eyes. She was shaking her head. A mighty death rattle rose from the throat of the tired holy man. *Let my people go!* he moaned. *Let my people go!*

On the pediatric ward, one of the nurses was cradling Eva in her arms. It was hard to believe that she was once more orphaned. It was our turn to throw a lifeline to a poor motherless child.

Although Eva's legal status as a ward of the court was clarified, no one knew what to do with her. Medically, she was ready to go home, but finding a foster home for her was a different matter. Most of the homes already had other children in them. Were we sure, they asked, that she was not contagious? Could we guarantee the foster mother that she would not get AIDS herself from washing and kissing her? The arguments went on, and Eva remained with us.

It was extraordinary how content she was, staying in her room when asked, without complaint. She did not cry to be embraced but was happy to be held when someone came to her. The child's life attested to the resilience of the human spirit.

We had no idea how long she could live. The nurses—now her mothers—began to decorate her room as if she would be with us for the rest of her life. A shag rug briefly relieved the hospital drab, but the infection-control people pressed for it to be removed. Someone bought Eva a little record player. She loved to play "Ghostbusters" and would invite us to come and dance with her. How she loved to dance! She made my afternoon rounds a joy.

Her chart became thick with so-called progress notes. *The patient is stable. The T4/8 ratio was remeasured and remains unaltered. Blood taken for febrile episode. No source of fever found.* There are many ways to say absolutely nothing.

Between the non-progress notes were intimations of the disaster that would ultimately come to pass. Our bright little daughter was losing her ability to walk and talk. She seemed unable to do things that she easily had done in the previous month. We were learning firsthand about the disastrous consequences of AIDS on the brain of a growing child.

It was during this time that the human immunodeficiency virus was first identified and a test developed. The staff all ran to be tested, most of us using numbers or pseudonyms rather than take the risk that someone might know if we were positive. No one who had cared for Eva had any evidence of the virus. The rules relaxed.

No one found a cure while she was in our care— or since. But progress of another sort did occur. As Eva continued to live on our ward, there was at first a subtle and later more obvious change in the way that decisions were made about her care.

No blood test was drawn, no medication ordered without consulting her nurses. A profound respect replaced the traditional turf wars between doctors and nurses. Any of the senior physicians who came along with a "bright idea" was quickly informed by the house staff that they would do nothing without consulting Eva's primary nurse.

❧   ❧   ❧

I was on call the last week of her life. For weeks the child's condition had been deteriorating, her liver riddled by an infection that poses no harm to healthy people. She did not leave her bed. As her tummy swelled to accommodate the tumor-like nodules, she refused to eat.

It was on a Sunday afternoon that one of the residents called me back to the hospital. It was obvious that Eva would die the same day. Legally, they needed a note written by the senior attending to let her pass without prolonging her misery.

DNR. Do not resuscitate. We had all agreed. The nurses would have it no other way, and they were right. But it was my voice that the state authorities must hear, my pen that must execute our final will and testament for our little daughter. Moments later, she passed from this life in her nurse's arms.

❧   ❧   ❧

That Sunday seems like a lifetime ago, as if AIDS has been with us forever. Today more than three hundred young children are under care in our hospital for the virus. In our pediatrics department, it is more common than cancer and far more deadly. But there has been progress for children with cancer, and I must believe that the legacy for the children of this new plague will follow.

Years ago, when I started to care for children with cancer, few survived. Neighbor children were sometimes forbidden by their parents to play with my patients with leukemia. It might be contagious by casual contact, mothers told their children. Fear does not demand facts.

Although there is no cure as yet, we are starting to see children with AIDS who are "long-term survivors." We dare to speak of it as a chronic disease. The legacy for the deadly virus's littlest victims will surely follow. That is how we began with cancer. First you survive with a disease, next you outlive it. But the first steps can be the loneliest of all.

Fortunately, these children do not walk alone. A consultant involved in Eva's care left his research laboratory to care for these children, day by day. The community has honored him for his dedication to patients with AIDS. "It's been good for him," his wife told me proudly. "It's been good for his soul."

Eva's primary nurse-mother left the in-patient ward to work full-time with children with AIDS. I hear her silver-bell voice in the clinic and see her eyes sparkle with love and hope as she greets and cares for each of these children.

The state responded to the crisis by developing an effective foster-care program. One woman retired from her nursing career to become a full-time foster mother who takes one child after another into her home and makes them welcome as long as they live. She lays one to rest, and then reaches out to the next.

Eva and LaVonne and Rahab were laid to rest so long ago, yet their legacy lives on through our lives. It is as if, with the child, Rahab passed a lifeline to LaVonne and through her, to us. And the lifeline will continue to be passed as long as there are those who are willing to hold out their hands to receive the precious gift.